28 Days to a New You

Anthony Harris is the author of *Your Body* (Prentice-Hall, Spectrum Books, 1982). He is the director of London's popular Keep Fit Studios and is acclaimed in England for his scientific research into vitamin C and female frame types.

28 Days
to a New You

A Complete Shape-Up Program for Your Whole Body

ANTHONY HARRIS

A SPECTRUM BOOK

Prentice-Hall, Inc., Englewood Cliffs, New Jersey 07632

Library of Congress Cataloging in Publication Data

Harris, Anthony B.
  28 days to a new you.

  "A Spectrum Book."
  Includes index.
  1. Reducing exercises.   2. Exercise for women.
3. Reducing diets.   I. Title.   II. Title: Twenty-eight
days to a new you.
RA781.6.H36   1983   613.7'1'088042   83-10953
ISBN 0-13-934794-1
ISBN 0-13-934786-0 (pbk.)

This book is available at a special discount when ordered in
bulk quantities. Contact Prentice-Hall, Inc., General
Publishing Division, Special Sales, Englewood Cliffs, N.J. 07632

10 9 8 7 6 5 4 3 2 1

ISBN 0-13-934794-1

ISBN 0-13-934786-0 {PBK.}

Production supervision and interior design
by Alberta Boddy
Manufacturing buyer: Doreen Cavallo
Cover design by Hal Siegel

Prentice-Hall International, Inc., *London*
Prentice-Hall of Australia Pty. Limited, *Sydney*
Prentice-Hall Canada Inc., *Toronto*
Prentice-Hall of India Private Limited, *New Delhi*
Prentice-Hall of Japan, Inc., *Tokyo*
Prentice-Hall of Southeast Asia Pte. Ltd., *Singapore*
Whitehall Books Limited, *Wellington, New Zealand*
Editora Prentice-Hall do Brasil Ltda., *Rio de Janeiro*

To my grandfather, Edward Barnard,
and my students past, present, and future.

Contents

Appendix 2 159

Preface

WELCOME TO THE PROGRAM

Through long experience, I have found that twenty-eight days is the average minimum time to change the shape of the figure. Accordingly, I have designed this course for the majority of women between the ages of 16 and 55 who are healthy but whose figures need more definition.

Together with the very best in nutritional and scientific workouts, this program presents an entirely new concept of figure development—pleasure. I am sure you will soon grasp its meaning as you work toward your new figure and see the truth of it in new vitality and mental awareness. Work steadily through the course day by day if you want the best results.

Good Luck,

Anthony Harris
London 1982

Acknowledgments

My thanks and admiration to the students and teachers (who were once my students) of the Anthony Harris Keep Fit Studios, for providing the living proof and realization of these new concepts in vitality and figure shaping.

28 Days to a New You

Day 1

HOW TO WORK THROUGH THE PROGRAM

This program is designed to meet the demands of ordinarily healthy women in the 16 to 55 age group. The program is corrective, progressive, and formative of the soft tissues on a skeletal frame that has reached its basically mature dimensions.

Twenty-eight days is the minimum time it takes most women to achieve their best figure. However, you can take longer if you feel it is more pleasant or convenient. Indeed, you can achieve excellent results and really learn about your own unique needs if you simply familiarize yourself with the program and then set a month aside for a dedicated effort.

Women of average build should follow the program as described. Women who are very slight, even skinny, should do all the exercises slowly. In general, this means adding two or three counts in the breathing sequences and doubling the relaxation times given in the protocols.

Women of heavier physique need to quicken the pace by taking off one to two counts in the breathing sequences and putting more effort into the exercises so they do them more quickly. They should also cut down relaxation times in the protocol by about half.

The ideal way to get your new figure is through advanced movement methods and improved eating habits. It is not necessary to weigh yourself early in the program. Don't worry about weighing yourself until you reach the topic in the course.

Work through each day's program. Progress will not accelerate if you try to do two day's work in one. Naturally, it may happen that circumstances may cause you to miss a day, in which case begin again at the last day you worked on the program. If you miss two days, go back two days, and so on.

Preprogram Preparation

A little care with choice of exercise wear beforehand will be beneficial to your comfort. In general, you need loose-fitting garments, no shoes, and nothing restrictive. Be careful of jewelry, hair pins, and brooches that can stick you. Check your exercise wear for large buttons, zippers, and anything that may press against your bones. If your exercise outfit does not measure up to these safety precautions, find one that does.

For general work, a leotard is suitable provided it is one of the zipless, buttonless, knot-less types. Leg warmers are also a good idea. However, because the exercises are done in privacy, you will find greater benefit in wearing as little as possible.

Always work out in a warm room without drafts. If necessary keep a sweater or sweatsuit available to keep warm when doing static relaxation work.

It is essential you work on a soft but firm surface. The support given by a thick pile carpet with underlay is excellent. The standard floor type used in our studio for these kinds of workouts is two layers of pile carpet on a wooden floor.

Daily Program Plan

Each day's work begins with a general introduction to the ideas and goals for that day's exercises. Following is a step-by-step introduction to the exercise, which you must follow exactly. This stage of the program is not doing the exercise, it is learning it, and the learning process is very much part of the program.

At this stage you work gently, patiently, and cautiously until you can do the exercise perfectly. In each exercise, there is much detail explaining what the exercise does and what to watch for when doing the exercise.

At the end of the exercise descriptions, a column under the heading of *Protocol* lists the exercises you have to do that day to fulfill the program requirements.

A good method of workout is to learn the exercises, and then have a break before coming to the Protocol section. In general, you should not do these workouts within two hours of a meal, and certainly never work out with a full stomach.

In Summary

I have found that students who are very unfit, but who are uninhibited and relaxed, do not suffer from soreness even after a strong workout, such as in Day 4 or 6. A relaxed, fun-seeking, but determined, approach is the best for figure work.

Even if you are very fit and already have a good figure, there is still a great deal for you to benefit from in the program concerning relaxation, body awareness, and shrewdly assessing your own body and your aims.

Experience has taught me that age is not a very useful criterion for assessing the promise of progress. Routinely, we see women in our studios in their late forties with bodies of thirty, and women in their twenties with bodies of thirty. Consequently, I have constructed the program so that no matter how good or poor a condition your figure is in, you can still improve it because the workouts use your body's mechanics and physiology. Therefore, the program is automatically and uniquely paced for each individual.

If you are pregnant, do not do the program. If you have recently given birth, check with your physician before beginning the program. If you have been under medical care, check with your physician before attempting the program. This program is based on the mechanics and physiology of the average healthy woman, and therefore should not be used by anyone else.

Men in the 16 to 55 age range can derive benefit from the course. Because of greater muscular mass and a difference in actual muscle fiber composition, the best physique program for men would have different emphases and exercises. However, the relaxation, stretching, and nutritional parts of the program are ideal. Men can use the course as a superb workout system, to improve fitness and weight levels, but they will not achieve the same shaping standards as women, for which the program is precisely designed.

The program is about vitality, self awareness, shape, and pleasure. If you enjoy it, you must be doing it right.

GOOD FIGURES

Over a period of ten years, in every class I took, in every seminar, in every new group of women I met, it was clear that there were always some women who others admired as being the possessors of make a good figure. Sometimes the woman was tall and slender, sometimes short and powerfully made, at other times of average dimensions, but always there were shared similarities that combined to make a good figure.

A good figure only happens when the muscles are strong enough to coordinate the skeletal frame in movement, so there is a natural grace in every movement the body makes. The lines of the body have an unmistakeable balance and elegance. There is a working wholeness about the limbs, the head, and the torso. When you see such a body, the face always expresses an appetite for and an enjoyment of life. Furthermore, a good figure is a *working* body. It can perform without stress or strain all the functions it is called upon to do in a normal working day and night.

A good figure is made up of health, grace, power, vitality, and naturalness. Your good figure will have all these qualities, but the result will still be unique. There will not be another like it in town or anywhere else.

STRETCHING

There are many stretching exercises in the program. The logic of stretching is as follows: The stretch is in the opposite direction to the wear and tear of the day. Research has shown that during the day the body builds fibrous material at points of maximum compression in an effort to meet the demands placed upon it. This leads to pain because nerves are pinched by the fibers, and also to poor muscle tone because the blood supplies are constricted.

By stretching in the reverse direction, the process of overfibering is slowed down. The effect of noncorrection is evident in the bowed back and broken lines of people's bodies who, merely in their fifties, have become inflexible.

PERSEPHONE (PER-SEF-OH-KNEE): Lie in the relaxed position shown in Figure 1.1, and place your hands in position. Exhale all the air from your lungs, and gradually breathe in as you smoothly stretch to the position in Figure 1.2. Hold your breath in the maximum stretch for a count of five, and then exhale with force as you relax back into the position in Figure 1.1. Again let the air naturally flow into your lungs. Now exhale completely, and begin the cycle again. Once you have coordinated these movements lying on your left side, turn to your right side and repeat the movements.

In the position in Figure 1.1, the knees are next to one another,

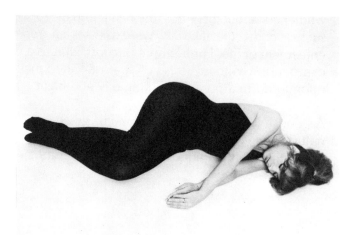

Figure 1.1

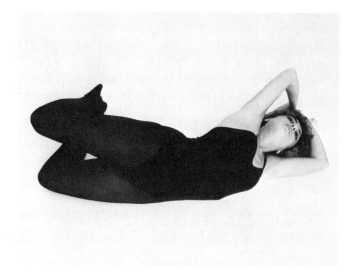

Figure 1.2

while in the position in Figure 1.2, they are apart, although the feet are still together. We have found that the arching of the torso and continuing the line of curve along the thighs causes the legs to automatically part at the knees. In other words, the position in Figure 1.2 is anatomically true. Also note how the arms are part of the large curve from the knees over the hips along the belly, up to the chest, and then on the underside of the arms.

FAT

The amount of body fat was more or less the same in all the women selected by other women as having the best figures. When we measured the fat percentage, we found it to be between 11 and 15 percent of the total body weight. Anything less, and the body was too thin, anything more, and the body was burdened with excess fat.

Excess fat is, as far as your real figure is concerned, *dead* tissue. It does not hold shape, it does no work for you, and it makes your heart work harder. The disadvantages of overweight actually go much deeper—being overweight cuts down your skin sensitivity, resulting in less sensual pleasure from touching and being touched. You also feel the air and the sun less.

Note we say excess fat. There is a best level of fat. Too much fat and you get the drawbacks, too little fat and other drawbacks occur. Not enough fat causes a lack of smooth body lines, a sunken face, and a feeling of discomfort in your own body movements because your bones bang and scrape too easily. You become oversensitive to heat and cold.

A figure deterioration of an extra ½ inch on the thigh is usually not so noticeable as it would be on the abdomen. The skin of the thigh is very elastic and tough and can maintain good contour even with an extra ½ inch on the thigh alone. Nevertheless, it is still better to remove it.

THINKING RIGHT ABOUT FAT

Currently, 40 percent of our energy needs come from fat, when it should be 15 percent. This excess fat intake means almost certain overweight. Furthermore, this is animal fat, which under human skin is usually hard, lifeless, and unpleasant to the touch. To have your best figure you need to cut down on animal fat. Cut out butter, ice cream, chocolate, hamburgers, sausages, french fries, potato chips, and fritters.

Good sources of fat, because other important nutrients are present, are fish, lean meat, cheese (not more than 3 ounces a day), plant margarine, nuts, vegetable oils, and whole-wheat bread.

There are many kinds of fats: Vegetable oils, such as safflower, wheatgerm oil, sunflower oil, contain *essential* fats, which are necessary as vitamins for good health. Use vegetable oils on salads and in cooking whenever you can. All varieties of fish are good sources of lecithins, an ingredient of skin, and a constituent of nervous tissue.

When you vary your fat intake, the fat and your skin changes from hard, cold, and lumpy, to soft, warm, and smooth. The effect on your looks and vitality should be profound.

FAT ASSESSMENT

To get the most out of the program, you must have standards to aim for, standards for your own physique.

Work through the following criteria and keep records so you can follow your progress.

Pinch Standards

I have found this simple method to be a reliable guide to the necessary amount of fat beneath the skin for a firm figure. Women with good figures, as judged by other women, have the following standards:

leg pinch	½ inch	(see #1.3)
thigh pinch	½ inch	(see #1.4)
tummy (abdomen) pinch	½ inch	(see #1.5)

In all, your *total* pinch (leg + thigh + tummy), should be 1½ inches, the sum of the three pinches.

You may find that your leg and thigh pinch is standard, but perhaps your tummy pinch is 1 inch. This is extremely common and usually means you are about 5 to 7 pounds of fat overweight.

Your weight need not necessarily fall by this amount during the program because you will be building muscle to contour your body.

Usually women in the 7 pounds overweight class lose their excess fat, in which case their pinch reaches the standard of 1½ inches. Because these women also put on about two to three pounds of muscles, their weight falls only by three to four pounds.

So, for a good figure, you need to reach the fat standards as determined by the pinch tests. Even if your weight stays the same, you will still look much trimmer and have a better body contour because you will have lost fat but built figure forming muscles.

If you have a standard ½ inch abdomen and lower leg pinch, but an inch or more at the thigh, the same points apply, but your weight excess is usually three to five pounds.

Leg Pinch

Sit as shown in Figure 1.3 and pinch the skin of your leg well below the knee. Make sure you get as big a pinch as you can, and measure it as shown in Fig. 1.3. The pinch shown is about ½ inch. Record your measurement in the box.

Thigh Pinch

Now stand up and deeply pinch your thigh, as shown in Figure 1.4. Measure the thickness of the pinch. In Figure 1.4 the pinch is about ½ inch. Record your measurement in the box.

Tummy Pinch

Deeply pinch your abdomen at the level of the navel but to one

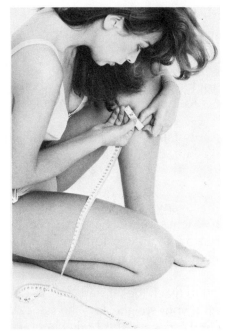

Figure 1.3

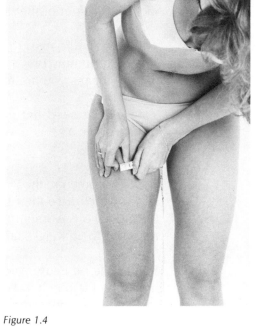

Figure 1.4

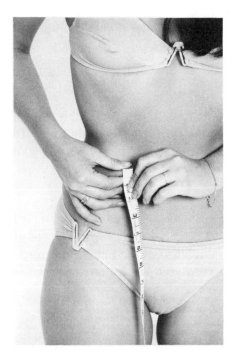

Figure 1.5

side as shown in Figure 1.5. Measure the thickness as shown in Fig. 1.5 where it is about ½ inch. Record your measurement in the box.

MY MEASUREMENTS

Leg Pinch

Thigh Pinch

Tummy Pinch

The ideal range is one to two inches. If this is your case, continue the program. If your pinch measurements adds up to more than 2½ inches, refer to Appendix One before continuing the program.

Day 2

BREATHING AND RELAXATION

The secret of good breathing is to work at breathing *out*. Most people breathe too shallowly so the blood does not receive as much oxygen enrichment as it should. Shallow breathing allows the waste material lactic acid to build up in the bloodstream. Excess lactic acid creates a feeling of anxiety. Aerobiosis, or good breathing, rids the body of this waste.

HELEN: Note the erect stance with the feet. Breathe in normally, and press your hands against your thighs as shown in Figure 2.1. Purse your lips as if you were going to whistle, and with a mental count of six, breathe out until your lungs are absolutely empty. At the same time, relax the pressure on your thighs. Let the air rush back in and repeat.

When you breathe in your tummy will swell out if you are relaxed, when you breathe out it will go back in.

Try this exercise in front of a mirror to check your progress.

PSYCHE (CY-KEY): Once you perfect Helen, you can explore the more advanced power of Psyche. In Psyche, it should be noted that the position in Fig. 2.3 is technically a strained position. Difficulty with this is never experienced because of an inhibited response, but because of muscular stiffness—and also in some cases because the tendons and muscles at the back of the leg are too short. There is little virtue in overstraining to reach this position, all that is needed is a minor feeling of making an effort.

The squat in Figure 2.2, however, can be accomplished by even very unfit people. Usually, there is no mechanical difficulty because this position ideally exploits the fine ball-and-socket-joints of the hip. Your back will find a welcome relief as you move your hips closer to your arms. When you get really good at it, you will find that your bottom almost touches the floor.

I hope you are beginning to see that there is a great deal to be learned about yourself in the quest for a better level of health in

Figure 2.1

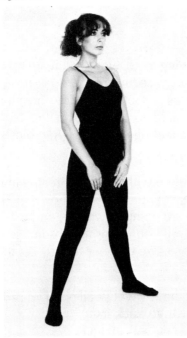

Figure 2.2

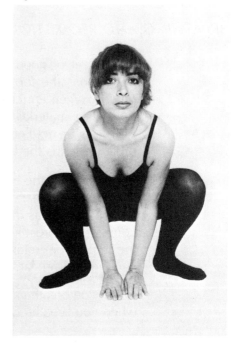

even the most simple movements. The movements in this program are anatomically true, and yet are as powerful as the most abstruse yogic or Zen exercises.

Simple movements account for 90 to 95 percent of the benefit in exercises, while difficult and outlandish movements only supply an extra five percent. The extra percentage employed by adept yogis is used to promote an extraordinary level of discipline. In this program I will show you how to develop a better body in twenty-eight days. For this purpose, I have chosen methods that deliver results commensurate with the effort and care you do them with.

Most women find a pleasant sensation of pleasure in the pit of the belly after a few cycles of Psyche. In some, waves of relaxation occur on the insides of their legs, up from the crotch over the abdomen to the breasts. These reactions are a sign your muscles and your lung movements are perfectly in tune.

The pleasure comes from the brain and solar plexus (a small "brain" in the front of the abdomen) producing endorphins—natural pleasure inducers and relaxers carried by the bloodstream.

This program is dedicated to such feelings of pure pleasure, because this pleasure is the result of good health. It may feel sexual, but it is not. The sad fact is that many people feel this pleasure only fleetingly, and then only for a fraction of time during sexual activity, hence they think the pleasure is sexual. It is more accurate to say that the pleasure of sexual feelings are part of the life force, not the other way around.

I emphasize the feeling of pleasure for two reasons. First, as I found in countless studio seminars, a majority of women quickly experience good feelings in their bodies by this simple exercise. Unfortunately, too high a proportion of them immediately proceed to inhibit these sensations. You can tell they do this because muscles that were relaxing and getting warmer are suddenly, by conscious effort, contracted—the classic inhibitive response. Now clearly, if you do exercises, you want the maximum benefit and the pleasure flow of the health flow, along with an increase in blood circulation and hormonal changes. Hence to inhibit it, to put it bluntly, is sheer ignorance of a basic body grammar.

The second reason for emphasis concerns the minority of women who are so tense and cut off from their bodies that they even find taking these positions difficult (especially the squat—an innocent posture which is mechanically correct for our skeletal structure, as shown in Figure 2.2).

With such dire tensions, pleasure and real, true, good health are impossible.

Consequently, if you are one of the majority, be glad, and encourage it.

If you are suffering an inhibitive response, think about what I have said and draw your own conclusion. Keep at the Helen and Psyche until you begin to experience what is your birthright.

Squat as shown in Figure 2.2, with your heels firmly on the ground, knees apart, and the palms of your hands pressed down. Look straight ahead with both hands placed firmly on the ground, and breathe normally a few times. Now purse your lips and blow air out gently until you experience a slight discomfort due to needing oxygen, and then let the air rush into your lungs as you stretch up to the position shown in Figure 2.3. Now that your lungs are fully filled, push the air out, keeping the position in Figure 2.3, and let the air come back in.

Do this exercise several times until you are breathing out for a count of ten, and breathing in—*letting* air in—for a count of five. When you become really proficient at this exercise, you will take five seconds to move from the position in Figure 2.2 to the position in Figure 2.3 (breathing in), and ten from the position in Figure 2.3 to the position in Figure 2.2 (breathing out).

PHAEDRA (FEE-DRA): Having worked through the two previous movements, now let's turn to a basic relaxed position, which is used many times in the 28-day program.

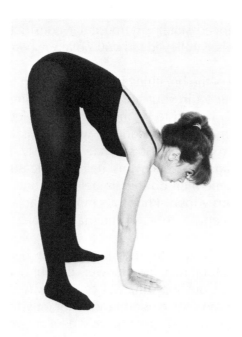

Figure 2.3

Phaedra is a very simple exercise, but as you get to know it better, you will find it has soothing powers. Gradually master the Phaedra breathing techniques, and subtly alter the Phaedra positions for a greater effect on you personally, and you should find that Phaedra is one of the cornerstones of the program. Long after the course you can still use Phaedra.

As you get better at Phaedra, you should find that your breathing becomes longer, and almost imperceptible. Furthermore, your belly will seem to cave in as the tensions in the pelvic floor, in the ribs, and in the large muscles of thighs and hips, dissolve as the endorphins do their work.

This exercise causes you to quiver because you reach a point (about one person in twenty find the quivering point nearer than 3 inches to the floor) where the opposing sets of muscles are exactly balanced. Like a tightrope walker, you have to constantly readjust your weight, except that your body does it automatically for you, so you quiver.

In this balanced state, any muscular constriction on nerves and blood vessels is relieved, so you obtain maximum sensitivity.

The rhythm of the breathing imparts a warmth to the pelvic floor, a sort of saucer set in your hip girdle. This feeling is often described as "sexual". It used to be thought that this feeling happened because the organs of the abdomen were being pressed rhythmically down onto the uterus and vagina. Obviously this is partially true, but men can also reach this relaxed, pleasurable condition in Phaedra. Some men do it extremely well and with great satisfaction. Obviously then, Phaedra's most essential nature is not pressure since men do not have internal genitalia.

The pleasure occurs through muscle tone because you have allowed the natural regulatory powers of your body to find their own way by consciously getting out of their way. Instead of clumsily flexing this and that muscle, and ignorantly tensing this and that part, in Phaedra you progressively educate yourself to stop mistreating yourself. The result is a wonderful sense of wellbeing.

Make sure you do Phaedra in entirely safe surroundings because the climax is usually a very deep sleep.

Assume the position shown in Figure 2.4. The arms are relaxed and lying at the sides. The back is resting on the floor with the legs wide apart.

Now raise your hips so that your bottom is about 3 inches from the floor. You can determine the distance by either looking in a mirror or feeling with your hand. Bring your feet back so you can just touch your heel with your fingertips. The left fingertips touch the left foot, and right fingertips touch the right foot. You should still have both legs wide apart with your knees facing outward.

Exhale gently for a count of ten, and then let the air flow back in for a count of five. Inhale and exhale gently without force—otherwise you will get a headache.

As you breathe this way, ease your hips by pressing your pubic arch up about half an inch at a time for one breathing in and out cycle. Move your feet and change the angle of your legs for greater comfort.

Eventually you reach a position in which you begin to quiver. You feel small oscillations of the spine, although some people have the same feeling in the knees.

Once you have found this point, stay there. Gently breathe as previously described, but put your arms over your head so they lie on the floor above your head.

You can reduce the quivering, not by inhibiting it (that would destroy the whole point) but by simply lowering your hips.

When you get tired, you can rest your hips on the floor.

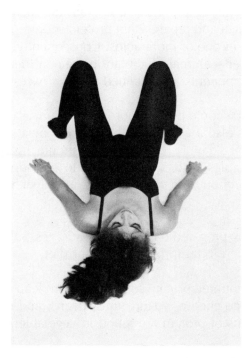

Figure 2.4

PROTOCOL

Helen: 3 minutes

Psyche: 20 x

Day 1 Protocol

Psyche: 20 x

Phaedra: 3 minutes

THINKING RIGHT ABOUT PROTEIN

Although protein is essential to the body, it does produce the toxic waste urea. Urea is lost through urine, and provided excessive protein is not eaten, the body is not harmed. There is a further problem in that not all proteins are equal. The animal proteins in eggs, meat, cheese, and fish all contain the materials the tissues need for growth and repair. Plant protein sources, such as cereals, are deficient in one or more acids. Consequently, protein sources must be mixed—animal plus plant protein. When mixed, all the essential components are obtained without excessive intake.

As a rule, you should not eat more than 4 ounces of meat or fish at a sitting. It is also a good idea to leave out meat and fish from at least one meal a day. Furthermore, you should always eat salads or boiled vegetables with protein meals to provide fiber and help mineral absorption from the protein, especially when the protein is meat.

Commercially prepared hamburgers, sausages, salamis, and pâtes are all too high in fat to be part of your diet.

Good, concentrated protein sources are fish, lean meat cuts, eggs, bacon, cottage cheese, yogurt, nuts, beans, and cereals. Weaker concentrations of protein are found in vegetables and fruits.

Boil, casserole, or grill your fish and meat, never fry. Eliminating frying reduces fat intake. Roasts are fine, but overlarge pieces (more than 2 pounds) do generate toxic materials more than grilling or boiling.

Day 3

BELLY SHAPING

The female body reveals its musculature through movement, or effort. The purpose of this program is to strengthen, shorten, and tone the muscles. Tailoring the muscle should ensure that the body is held together in the manner its structure demands. This is what is meant by a good figure, and a good figure cannot be obtained without power.

Within your own particular skeletal frame, your muscles have to reach a certain tone and power to give you the figure you should have—not someone else's figure, but your own.

Stereotyping the female figure is merely ignorance, and ultimately leads to a restricted view of natural health and power. Nevertheless, all women need to train their muscles to a standard for their frame so the frame can be held properly, move well, and meet the demands of life.

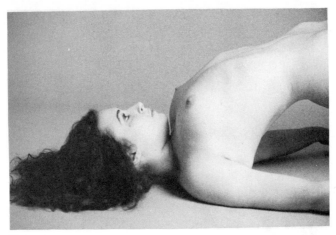

Figure 3.1

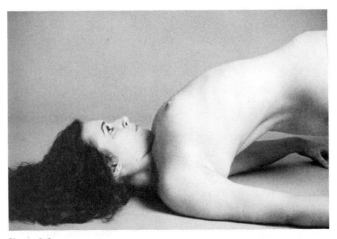

Figure 3.2

The relationship between body contours and muscle can be seen by studying Figures 3.1, 3.2, and 3.3.

In Figure 3.1 a professional dancer reveals abdominal muscles, indicating the structure of the abdomen (see same position in Aphrodite, Figure 3.5). The abdomen has valleys at the hip bones that rise in the center where the long abdominal muscles connect the pubic arch to the ribs. Note how the rib bones stick out. The body twisted in this position (Figure 3.2) reveals the work being done by strong muscles along the spine. The erector muscles along the spine are essential for a good posture and a well-shaped waist.

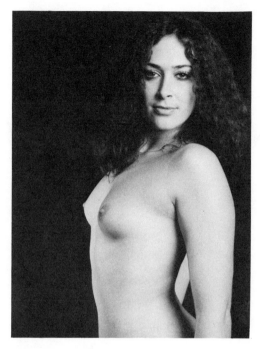

Figure 3.3

Also notice the economy of effort; As there is no excess force on the hand, it is entirely relaxed with the pressure being borne by the top of the back, the upper arms, and the feet.

Figures 3.1 and 3.2 reveal bone and muscular structure, but when the body is relaxed (Figure 3.3), there is no sign of these powerful elements of the physique. Indeed, even in a powerful female body able to perform the extremes of physical exertion in a graceful manner, such as a dancer's body, the relaxed muscles are not "cut" out from the rest of the body.

APHRODITE (AFRO-DIE-TEA): Take the relaxed position as shown in Figure 3.4. Breathe in as you gently push your back up to the position in Figure 3.5. Hold your breath for a count of three, and push the air out as you come back to the position in Figure 3.4. Breathe in, as you ascend again to the position in Figure 3.5. Breathe out as you come down. Practice until you have a coordi-

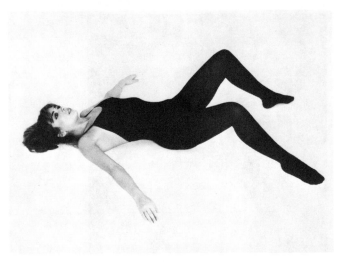

Figure 3.4

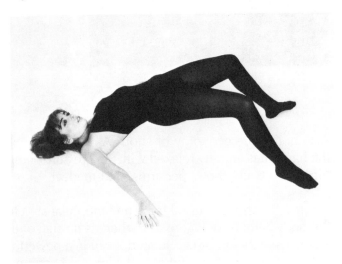

Figure 3.5

nated rhythm, gently pressing up with your feet in a steady manner with no jerking, and pushing air out and letting it come back of its own accord.

Having accomplished this at the top of the ascent, twist your hips to the right and then to left. Then descend from the middle position as shown in Figure 3.2. These are merely introductory exercises to Aphrodite, which is now performed fully as follows.

24

Lie as in Figure 3.4, and steadily breathe in on a count of five, so you are fully inhaled at the position in Figure 3.5. Hold this position for a count of three, and then exhaling steadily, consciously push the air from your lungs in a steady stream. Simultaneously, twist to the right, to the left, and then back to the middle position. Still exhaling, descend to the position in Figure 3.4 again. The exhalation should take twice as long as breathing in. When you are adept, you will do this with a rise and inhalation of five seconds, an exhalation and a twist and then a descent of altogether ten seconds.

The effect is to exercise not only your back, thighs, arms, and lungs, but also your abdomen.

Now set up a mirror so you can watch yourself doing Aphrodite. Concentrate on performing it as strongly, smoothly, and gracefully as you can, meanwhile observing the anatomical points already mentioned.

Watch your thigh muscles and the way your chest moves.

As you become more adept, rise on the balls of your feet, but always work hard on the line from your knee to abdomen. To remove stress from the back, pull the abdomen in as you ascend. This will also make you work even harder because you will be using your tummy muscles against the incoming air.

PROTOCOL

Aphrodite: 20 x, without rest, build to a rhythm, and keep it. When you have finished 20, lie relaxed in the position in Figure 3.4, and concentrate on your breathing cycle.

Helen: 3 minutes

Psyche: 20 x

Day 1 protocol

Psche 20x

Phaedra: 3 minutes

You need carbohydrates for a clean energy source. I say "clean," because your body burns carbohydrates smoothly and quickly to produce energy for all vital processes without making difficult-to-handle waste products.

You can only store enough carbohydrates to run a marathon. If you take more carbohydrates than you need in a day, your body cannot burn it but changes it to fat, which is deposited around your soft organs internally, and under your skin.

For good health, the best sources of carbohydrates are those that also give fiber. Fiber is a carbohydrate too, but is indigestible and cannot give you energy. The function of fiber is to exercise the 27 feet of food canal from mouth to anus. Without fiber, this large system becomes slack, resulting in poor figure lines at the belly and waist and the likelihood of impaired health.

Good sources of quick energy and fiber are fresh fruits and vegetables. Skimmed milk powders provide carbohydrates but no fiber. Honey and molasses are concentrated, and good energy sources. The importance of fruit is that its natural sugars (not table sugar) are absorbed quickly into the bloodstream without digestion, so energy availability is quick, while little digestive energy is expended.

Your digestive system is designed for the fruit and vegetable carbohydrates in the fiber-water structure of these natural foods. The large amounts of white table sugar eaten by many women presents a difficulty in making large amounts of the enzyme sucrase to digest it. This is an enforced or stressful response of your body, one it was not designed for.

Sugar then cannot form part of an optimum way of life. Your progress in the next 28 days will be greater if you do not eat any more sugar. This means you must look at food labels to see if sugar has been added. Looking at labels is essential because you will find corned beef and most canned soups and stews have sugar added to them. Pickles also contain sugar but since these are only a relish or garnish, they can be taken. It is only the bulk foods that contain sugar you need to avoid.

If you have a sweet tooth, use honey in your coffee, or tea. You will find you need less than sugar. Sweeten cereals with any kind of fresh fruit. You can eat as much fiber as you like. Similarly, vegetables, rather than pastries should bulk out your food.

Arranging Your Meals

You must eat a proper breakfast. If you do not, your blood glucose level will fall, so that by 10 or 11 A.M. you will have a headache. Most obese people miss breakfast. A minimal breakfast is as follows.

Whole wheat cereal is an excellent source of fiber. With more people returning to natural foods, many varieties are on the market. Skimmed milk or fruit (apples, oranges, bananas, pears, grapefruit, and so on) followed by a small protein course (such as grilled bacon with the fat cut off after grilling) are basic and delicious. A small poached or grilled fish, or one of three weekly eggs (poached or boiled) are also good sources. Garnish with any fresh or grilled vegetables you like. Tea or coffee, fresh fruit or vegetable juice complete your breakfast. At breakfast you may eat as much as you like within these rules.

How to Improve Your Eating

To get the best results in this program, you need to eat *variedly, freshly,* and *often.* As the program expands, you will understand why but start applying these principles today.

Varied Eating
You should eat:

> some meat and/or fish daily,
> some fresh vegetables daily,
> some green vegetables daily,

some citrus and other fruits daily,

some whole grain cereals daily,

some whole grain bread daily,

some milk, some cheese, some yogurt daily,

some beans and/or lentils daily,

about two to three eggs a week,

4 ounces of liver each week.

Cut out carbonated drinks, potato chips, hamburgers, peanut butter, ice cream, sweets, and confections.

Fresh Eating
Eat fresh meat, fish, vegetables, fruits, and nuts. Also eat unrefined cereals and bread. Keep canned and frozen foods to a minimum.

Eating Often
Eat breakfast and a snack at 11 A.M.—fruit is a good idea. Eat lunch and a 4 P.M. snack—fruit again. After a meal you should never feel bloated.

Further Methods for Improving Your Nutrition

Reduce your Fat Intake by
—cooling soups and stews so that the fat rises and skim it off with a ladle,

—grill instead of roast, grill instead of frying,

—cut off fatty portions of meat after cooking (totally fatless meat will not cook well).

Increase your Fiber Intake by
—eating fresh fruit and vegetables,

—eating whole grain bread and cereals.

Shopping

DON'T BUY	BUY
Sugar	Fruit juice, fresh fruit, dried fruits
Cream	Milk, skimmed milk

DON'T BUY	BUY
Full-fat cheese	Low fat, cottage cheese
Roasted and salted nuts	Fresh nuts, nuts in the hull
Chocolate	Use cocoa powder, fruit

Buy Fresh Dairy Foods

—Use Unhomogenized fresh milk and discard some of the cream.

—Cheese of the low fat variety (1–3 ounces a day), or traditional variety (1 ounce a day).

Buy Unprocessed, Whole Grain Cereals

—Cracked wheat, rolled oats, rice, millet, barley, corn, wheat, oats, rye flakes

—Whole grain biscuits and bread

—Whole grain pastas

—Sunflower seeds, sesame seeds.

Buy Fresh Fruit and Vegetables

—Dried fruit

—Dried beans, pulses, lentils

Buy Meat, Fish, Poultry

—Obtain fresh from butcher

Buy Fresh Sea Foods

Restaurants

Choose the best restaurant you can afford, and then apply the rules you have already learned to the menu. Look for grilled foods, not those roasted or fried. Choose a salad, not a buttered vegetable.

Day 4

WAIST AND THIGHS

Today stretching and hard work are the emphasis for the waist and thighs. We will be using three exercises; Iris, Ariadne (arri-ad-knee), and Artemis (ar-tea-miss).

IRIS (Figures 4.1–4.3): This exercise is designed to strengthen the back, especially along the spine. As you get better at it, pull your abdomen in as you blow air out. Make sure you press your body weight onto the ground by your heels and not on your toes. If you can't do it at first with your feet flat on the floor, do it very slowly, gradually easing your body into the right position.

Keep your knees out as far as possible, thereby stretching the inside of the thigh. Iris increases circulation at the crotch and top of the thighs (especially the inner areas) thereby helping to mobilize fat excess. Iris also strengthens the muscles underneath the breasts and helps in uplift. There is also a shortening of waist muscles, which leads to an improved waist line. When you become really proficient, widen your legs still further, and squat even deeper.

Begin by standing as shown in Figure 4.1. Purse your lips and blow air out as you spread your legs and raise your arms to the position in Figure 4.2. Let the air come back naturally into your lungs.

Now push the air out, as you fall with the weight of your body on your heels to the position in Figure 4.3.

Make sure your back is held straight and your arms kept up.

Push hard on your heels as you breathe in to ascend to the position in Figure 4.2 again.

Now push the air out as you lower to the position in Figure 4.3 again.

Repeat exercise several times until you are able to do it in a controlled manner.

ARIADNE (ARRI-AD-KNEE): Starting from the position in Figure 4.1, stretch your arms above your head, and grasp the first two fingers of your right hand. Pull strongly as you twist your hips in large circles (Figure 4.4) 10 times in one direction, then 10 times in the opposite direction.

As you do so, you will find that your breath is pumped naturally in and out.

Once you have mastered the movement slowly, circle back to the right and left, and forward as far as you can.

Ariadne is a waist shaper, and teaches you how to control the massive thigh muscles as you move on the ball and socket joints of the thighs. When you can do Ariadne, then you can change fingers on each revolution. You will immediately feel the effect on your frame of the pull on the fingers.

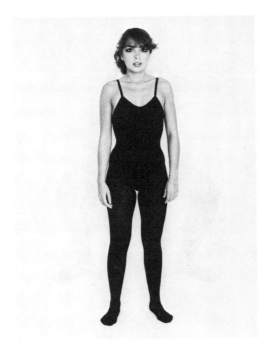

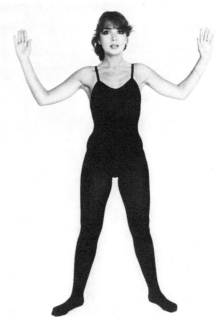

Figure 4.1

Figure 4.2

Figure 4.3

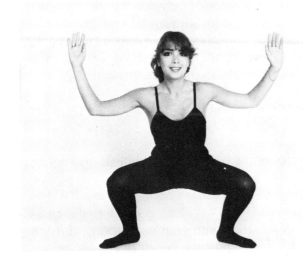

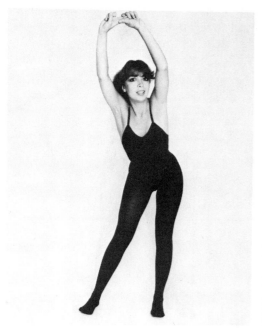

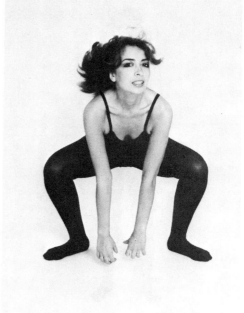

Figure 4.4

Figure 4.5

The stronger you pull your fingers in this movement (Figure 4.4), the more work is done by your muscles between the ribs. You not only improve their tone, but also improve your skin quality. As you get to know this exercise, pull your abdomen in as you circle back, and let it out as you come forward. At the same time, breathe in as you circle back, and breathe out as you come forward.

ARTEMIS (AR-TEA-MISS): Artemis has a strong shaping effect on the back of the thigh and top of the thigh.

The large bottom muscles of the buttocks, the gluteals also get an excellent work-out.

Starting from the position in Figure 4.1, leap gently into the air as you spread your legs, descending with your upper body to reach the position in Figure 4.5, while pushing the air out as you do so.

From the position in Figure 4.5 breathe in as you leap back to the position in Figure 4.1 again.

Try this sequence out slowly at first until you have determined you can do the movement in a controlled manner.

Once you have coordinated the movements, leap up from the position in Figure 4.5 as high as you can and bring your legs together. As you reach the highest point, open your legs as you come down to the position in Figure 4.5 again.

When you do this well, you will land without a jolt, or without much noise, because you come down on the ball of your foot, and then onto your heel, all in a split second.

PROTOCOL

Iris: 10 x
Ariadne: 10 x clockwise, 10 x counterclockwise
Phaedra: 1 minute (Day 2)
Artemis: 20 x
Iris: 5 x
Ariadne: 3R x, 3L x
Artemis: 5 x
Iris: 5 x
Ariadne: 5R x, 5L x, Very slowly, until you are almost stationary

Protocol Day 3
Phaedra: 1 minute (Day 2)

BALANCED EATING

By now you should be eating greater varieties of protein, along with a good balanced breakfast and four small meals a day.

As you can see from Table 4.1, eating more protein, fruits, and vegetables, increases fiber and decreases fat. Eating more cereal products, bread, and unsugared breakfast cereals gives a balance of protein, fat, fiber, and carbohydrates. Observe too, how a diet too reliant on protein has very little fiber.

If you haven't yet begun to use whole grain cereals, brown instead of white bread, wholewheat instead of white bread, begin as soon as possible.

TABLE 4.1. Average Percentage Composition of Common Foods

	% PROTEIN	% CARBOHYDRATE	% FAT	% FIBER
Cereals	11	15	5	10
Cakes, Pies, Puddings, Biscuits	6	53	10	4
Milk	3	5	4	0
Egg and Cheese Dishes	10	15	30	0
Meat, Poultry, Fish	23	Effectively 0	14	0
Meat, Fish, Poultry Product Dishes	10	10	12	3
Fresh Vegetables, Fruits	2 (Beans higher)	11	0*	5
Nuts	10	10	30	7
Sugar	0	100	0	0

*Except Soya Beans
© Dr. Anthony Harris, 1983.

Day 5

SEX AND YOUR FIGURE

Healthy intercourse is a ballet of coordination. To gain as much from intercourse as possible, your body must be healthy.

Most human intercourse occurs in the missionary position. This frontal position is excellent for the figure.

There has been a great deal of speculation concerning the inadequacy of the missionary position. Much interest has been shown in various other positions, some of them athletic and some just plain uncomfortable. Standing up usually results in weak knees. Although a woman on all fours entered from behind is mechanically satisfactory, face-to-face contact is reduced and can cause a sense of loneliness. Actually, the face-to-face and chest-to-chest contact, as well as the back support of the missionary position for women, make this position uniquely human.

If during intercourse, your partner is merely being used as a vehicle for your sexual pleasure and satisfaction, your own satisfaction and pleasure are diminished. The two bodies only fully flower in tandem.

Being a passive sex object shortchanges both partners.

If only the genitalia are involved with sex, alienation is always a danger. Kissing each other's eyes, mouth, cheeks, and forehead all are possible in the missionary position, while at the same time allowing entire genital contact.

The penis can enter the woman's vagina shallowly or deeply, softly or vigorously, and press or not press against the clitoris. The woman can be just as forceful in her pelvic movements as the man. Her feet splayed but firmly on the ground allows her back to arch up and come down as she feels necessary, all with the movements of her lover. She can also control his movements by her gestures, speaking, touch, and the powerful clasp of her thighs.

The male's chest is unimpeded, unless he is lying full weight on top of the woman, so breathing can be deep. The heart does not have to pump blood up against gravity, so circulation is free. The top of the shoulders and feet can carry the weight, so lovers can arch and flex their spines, pull in their abdominal muscles, and twist a little. All these are basic strengthening and shaping movements of the body.

Accordingly, many of my exercises (some of which are in this program) are based on the uninhibited health-enhancing movements of the female body during satisfactory intercourse. *What we found was that the sense of pleasure is actually inherent in the movements of intercourse even without any sex occurring.*

We have therefore discovered a uniquely enriching principle. Active sexuality confers an improved body, and an improvement of the body confers better sex. One helps the other and improvement goes together.

This is the active principle of the relationship between sex and health. However, there is also the passive principle, where once the flow of pleasure is in full flood, you turn off all muscular tenseness that might impede it. Hence, healthy sexual intercourse has periods in it where there is little movement but the charge of bliss and satisfaction is at a height. Consequently, I have also developed exercises to reach this stage of pleasurable health. (For example, see Phaedra, Day 2).

VENUS (VEE-NUS): Venus shapes the groin, inner thighs, and belly but its other bonus is the way it deeply relaxes the whole body, thereby increasing circulation and muscle tone. It is also useful as a means of reducing menstrual cramps when used regularly.

Lie on your back, raise your arms over your head, and let them lie totally relaxed as shown in Figure 5.1.

Bend your legs at the knees, and place the soles of your feet together, keeping the feet on the floor.

Let your legs separate under their own weight, so that you lie perfectly relaxed as shown in Figure 5.1.

Figure 5.1

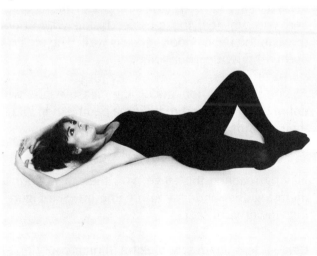

You should not feel a sense of tension in your legs, so move until you find the most relaxed position.

Lie in this position as you push the air out through your mouth with pursed lips for a count of ten. Let the air flow back in of its own accord.

Continue breathing in this way until you are exhaling completely, in which case the flow of air out will take about 15-20 seconds, and the flow of air back in (also through your mouth) will take about five seconds.

When you begin to feel a pleasurable sensation in your tummy and on the inside of your legs, you are ready for the next part of the exercise.

As you breathe in, press your feet together with increasing pressure. As you exhale, gradually release the pressure.

Get into the rhythm where you press your feet, breathe in, relax your feet, and breathe out.

When you are adept at this exercise, you will find that you receive increasingly pleasurable pulses of feeling up your thighs and up the front of your belly. These pulses will become more rhythmic, and you will feel the muscles inside your abdomen, especially those in the pelvic floor, relax as well. The pleasure will be greater and will flow up your spine.

As you become more adept, the pleasure flow will spread up your entire body to your throat. Some people then increase the tempo of their rhythm, while others do not. Your tempo is entirely a matter of what is most beneficial to you.

Having reached this stage, you then raise your feet as you press them together and as you breathe in. (See Figure 5.2.) On exhaling, lower your feet.

Once adept, gradually breathe in on a count of ten, and gradually increase the force with which you push your feet together as

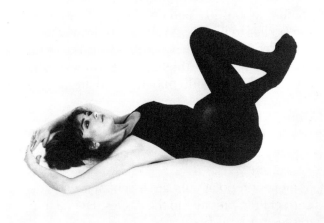

Figure 5.2

shown in Figure 5.2. Then blow the air out and gradually decrease the pressing of your feet until you reach the position in Figure 5.1 and there is a zero pressure. Begin the exercise all over again.

When you have coordinated this exercise, you can go on to higher levels of relaxation by pulling in the abdomen as in Figure 5.2, and pressing your feet and curving your hips up, so they come off the ground. You will only be able to keep the position for a very short time with completely filled lungs. When you tire, let the air out and descend as previously described.

THINKING RIGHT ABOUT MINERALS AND TRACE ELEMENTS

Minerals

Much lowered vitality can be traced to excessive sodium intake and too little intake of trace elements. Minerals and trace elements must be in the right proportions in our bodies. Much energy has to be expended if the diet is unbalanced in correcting the inadequate mineral and element levels. However, the diet you are working toward is far superior in mineral balance than the average Western diet.

41

Sodium
Most fresh vegetables, fruits, and untreated meats are very low in sodium (about .01 percent weight for weight) and about right for our bodies to handle. Many foods have added salt, such as cheese (1 percent), bacon (1 percent), salted butter (.5 percent). Shellfish, however, are quite high in salt in the fresh, untreated state (.2 percent), but provide minerals and are included in your diet.

Corned beef can approach 2 percent by weight in sodium, and whole, processed beef extracts are also very rich in salt.

Potassium
Sodium and potassium are essential for nervous coordination, and correct fluid pressure in the tissues. Hence, mineral balance affects the feel of your body.

Nuts, vegetables, and fruits, which are poor sources of sodium, are moderate sources of potassium (about .3 percent), while bread contains about twice as much sodium as potassium. While this is acceptable for good health, in order to help this balance you need to eliminate excessive salt from your diet.

Chloride
The chief function of chloride is to balance sodium and potassium, as well as calcium. Both sodium and potassium are found as chlorides in food, so the sources of chloride are those of potassium and sodium. Balanced amounts are found in fresh food.

Calcium
Good dietary sources for calcium are cheese (as high as .7 percent), milk, beans, nuts, and bread because calcium salts are added to it. A good figure depends on calcium because the body's shape is partially controlled by the skeleton.

Phosphorus
Approximately 80 percent of your phosphorus is present in your bones. Phosphorus is an essential element made of several molecules that facilitate energy release from carbohydrates. Other phosphorus compounds store chemical energy. As a general rule,

a diet with dairy produce and meat is adequate in calcium and phosphorus.

Magnesium
Magnesium is essential in the energy release from food. It is found in chlorophyll, the green pigment of plants. Fresh green vegetables are essential for vitality.

Sulphur
Sulphur is obtained from proteins and used to make the proteins of skin and hair, as well as all other proteins in the body.

Iron
More than 50 percent of iron in the body is found in hemoglobin, the red pigment in red blood cells that carry oxygen. Menstrual blood loss is a significant depletion of iron reserves.

Too little iron in the body causes lassitude, and it is a common condition among women of child bearing age. Ten percent of women in Great Britain and the United States are affected. Green vegetables, meat, and salads are important in a diet aimed at vitality and vigor. Green vegetables are not only a source of iron, but they also provide vitamin C. Eat an orange after your steak and salad.

Trace Elements

Iodine
Most of the iodine needed is used to make the hormone thyroxine, which is crucial for regulating energy. It is made in the thyroid gland in the neck.

Adequate sources of iodine are seafoods, iodized salt, and vegetables grown on iodine-rich soil.

Fluorine
The most common source of this mineral is treated drinking water (but less than three parts per million), where it is present as fluoride, not fluoro-additives. Its presence reduces tooth decay.

Cobalt
Cobalt is an essential part of vitamin B_{12}, which will be discussed later.

Copper
Your body uses copper to help make its hemoglobin.

A wide variety of foods provides adequate copper, but processing of food (the polishing of rice and the whitening of wheat flour) reduces the level of available copper.

Above certain concentrations, copper salts are extremely poisonous, so supplements are not acceptable.

Manganese
Found throughout the tissues of the body, manganese helps in removing waste products of normal bodily functions.

Chief sources are cereals, although nuts and beans also supply important amounts.

Zinc
Zinc is involved in sexual function and is essential. It also helps in cleansing the blood of respiratory waste.

Mixed diets provide between 10 to 15 mg a day, but this is increased by two or more fold when whole grains, fish, and meat are eaten.

Other Trace Elements

Selenium is closely allied with vitamin E. The metal molybdenum is found in many human enzymes and is essential. Nickel, also a metal, is part of many enzymes.

There are other trace elements, as yet not understood, so we need to have a fresh and raw diet, especially in unprocessed grains, to be sure of getting what we need for good health.

Mineral Requirements
for Health, Looks, and Vitality

We require between 2-5 gms of sodium chloride a day, more if excessive sweating occurs because cramps and muscular weakness can arise through a lack of sodium. These quantities are exceeded greatly in Western diets, but can be maintained by a mixed, varied diet. Potassium needs are much less and are easily met by a mixed diet.

Iron requirements are usually fixed at 18 mg for still menstruating women, and 18 mg for pregnant and lactating women.

Calcium requirements are set at 650 mg a day. Table 5.1 shows average food contents. Observe how we rely on high-protein foods for iron and dairy produce for calcium.

TABLE 5.1. Average Iron and Calcium in Common Foods (in mg of mineral per 3–4 ounces of food)

	IRON	*CALCIUM*
Cereals, Cereal Products	2	100
Cakes, Pies, Puddings, Biscuits	1	100
Milk	.05	120
Eggs, Cheese Dishes	.7	150
Meat, Poultry, Fish	1.8	25
Meat, Poultry, Fish Dishes	1.5	40
Vegetables	.8	40
Fruits	.5	15
Nuts	2	40

© Dr. Anthony Harris, 1983

Magnesium requirements are approximately half of that of calcium; diets rich in calcium will also generally be adequate in magnesium.

Zinc and copper are generally adequate in fresh mixed foods.

Approximately .1 mg of iodine is required daily. Because salt is used in cooking, seasalt, which contains iodine, is preferable to noniodized table salt.

PROTOCOL

Venus: 10 x

Day 4 Protocol

Venus: 10 x

Phaedra: 2 mins (Day 2)

Day 6

THIGHS

Except for a minority, most women's thighs are in poor shape. The thigh line seen from the side is usually good with high heels on, but this is artificial and temporary.

Thigh muscles are among the strongest in the body, but despite all the standing women do, they seldom squat, sit with their legs apart, and rarely lie with the legs higher than the body. Together with high heels, this leads to deterioration of your natural thigh line.

The muscles must be strong enough to form the thigh line by their natural shape pushing up against the skin. Hence, you need powerful exercises to increase the blood flow in your muscles.

The thigh line is also spoiled by excess fat at the top, back, and inside top of the thigh. Naturally, there is a gap at the top near the crotch, the crotch gap, and you should be able to see through it even with the legs together. When I say *should*, I mean that is the thigh *design*. The thigh bones are set at an angle wide enough apart for there to be a crotch gap. The crotch gap is seldom found in men.

The skin of a healthy thigh has a sheen at the front and a rougher quality at the sides and back. The inside of the thigh is usually smoother than silk. If your distribution isn't like this, check during the next few weeks because it usually improves quickly during the program.

Caucasian and black women have longer legs than oriental and hispanic women, and so tend to find the exercises below more difficult, while women with shorter legs need to improve the speed of movement to make sure they get a workout.

Things to Do

Watch young girls playing and observe how they squat. It is not uncommon for women, even in their late teens, to have lost this ability. Relearn it. Crossing your legs will eventually lengthen one leg and spoil your gait—avoid crossing your legs.

When a woman is entirely relaxed, her legs splay. Some behaviorists mistake this for body language implying a sexual come-on. It is not. The way women have to imprison their bodies in stereotypic rigid postures is archaic and ignorant. It is a pity some scientists mistakenly reinforce these prejudices by confusing learned roles with natural ones. The legs in men and women naturally splay when sitting relaxed by reflex on the buttock muscles. You have to force your knees together and this can be proved by measuring the tension of inner thigh muscles. For healthy legs, sit easy. Whenever possible, put your feet up, to take the hydraulic pressure off your veins.

You recoat your legs with new skin many times a year. Slough off the old skin by rubbing *up* from your feet with a strong sponge or washcloth without soap. Soap can be used afterwards, but not in excess because soap removes oils from the skin.

Doing really hard exercise, it is remarkable how your mind is stripped of its preoccupations with your own image. You begin to see yourself clearly and accurately. This effect is heightened the harder you work. It is as if the body, basically honest, at last gets through to an uncluttered area of the mind. Psychologically, the phenomenon is a kind of displacement, whereby the effort of working your body enables you to bypass habits of thought and discover truer perceptions. The value of seeing yourself truly is immeasurable, because once you have that perceptive ability, you can use it (simply tune in to the circuit you have discovered) on other people and see them clearly too.

When you become fatigued, you cannot watch yourself as well (at least, beginners in body lore will find this, adepts enter even clearer mental processes the more fatigued they become). At this point, you have to activate your will. The automatic power of the body is limited, but when directed by will, it extends considerably. This is one of the reasons why so many artists (singers, dancers) and athletes appear to have quite ordinary physiques but exceptional powers—they use their will.

ATHENA (AH-THEE-NA): Lie on your back, with your hands firmly placed palms down by your sides as shown in Figure 6.1. Breathe in as you raise your legs. Reach back with your legs to touch the ground behind your head (see Figure 6.2), then breathe out as you flick them quickly forward, *stopping them about a foot from the floor.* Lower your legs gently, and then start the exercise over again. You may find you have to open your legs to do it. When you flick your legs forward, you will have to push hard on your hands to stop the descent of your legs properly. Keep your head down. This exercise is a very fine tummy shaper.

BRISEIS (BRI-SEE-IS): Once you have coordinated these movements, stay in the position in Figure 6.3, letting your knees sink toward your body. Many women easily allow the knees to come to rest on either side of the head. Breathe naturally in this position. If you are doing the exercise properly, you will find this a very soothing and relaxed position. Relax your bottom.

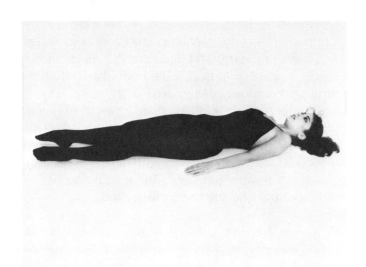

Figure 6.1

Figure 6.2

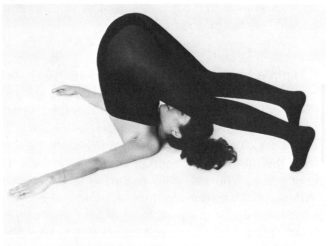

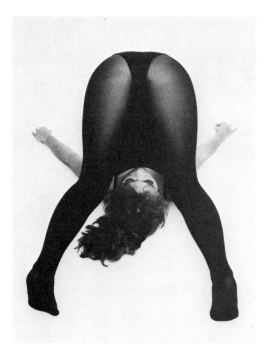

Figure 6.3

CALLISTO (CAL-LISS-TOE): Do this exercise very gently at first and never on a slippery floor. Make sure as you stretch out you pull your tummy in. Assume the position in Figure 6.4, thighs vertical. Facing directly ahead, slide your hands along the floor and push them far from you, while *gradually* unfolding your body. Stop sliding when your spine is in a bow shape downward as in Figure 6.5. Find the position you can hold without consciously flexing any muscles. Maintain the position for 15 seconds while breathing naturally. Then, pull yourself back to the starting position in Figure 6.4, using your tummy and leg muscles.

Once you have the basic movement, begin with your knees as far apart as possible and creep on the floor with your hands to the point in Figure 6.5, gradually exhaling as you do so. (A count of five to do this is adequate), now breathe in as you return to the position in Figure 6.4, taking a count of five to complete the movement. Callisto is excellent for allowing the breasts to flush with blood and lymph.

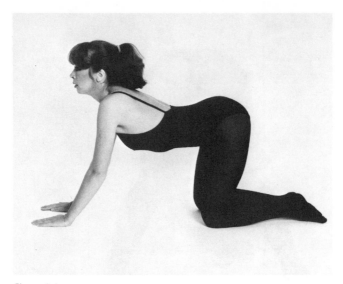

Figure 6.4

Figure 6.5

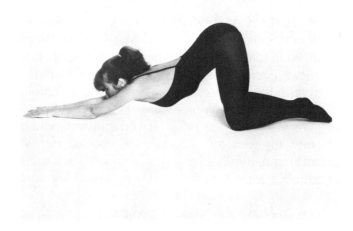

CASSANDRA (CAH-SAND-DRA): Sit on the floor with your legs straight out in front of you. Put your hands behind you with the fingers pointing in the opposite direction to your legs and rest the weight of your back upon your hands. Now raise your entire body up on your toes, forming a bridge. Let your head hang as in Figure 6.6. From this position, *gently* stretch up as you push your pubic arch up. *Do not strain*. Now relax so that you almost touch the ground with your bottom and then push back up again. Breathe in as you go up, out as you come down.

This exercise can only be done properly if there is a firm basis of support with the palms of the hands, and the shin-bones are vertical when you are in the bridge position. It is also quite important to have your legs about 18 inches to 2 feet apart, so that there is just a slight discomfort in the width of spread.

As you get better, increase the spread of your feet more.

Cassandra clearly strengthens the back, but as you spread the legs wider, more and more work is done on the inside of the thighs.

Figure 6.6

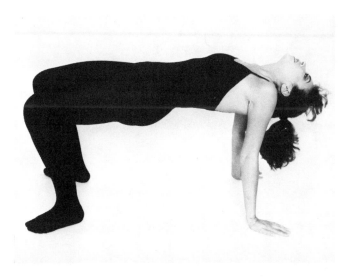

<u>NYMPH:</u> Nymph strengthens the front of the body and shapes the small of the back.

Start by lying on your tummy and putting your arms out on either side in a crucifix position, making sure the palms of both hands are firmly on the floor. Keep your shoulders to the ground and look up. (See Figure 6.7.) Bend your left leg at the knee until it is about vertical, point your toe, and move your leg over your other leg so that the knee touches the ground as far as you can as in Figure 6.8. But do keep your shoulders in contact with the ground. If you find this exercise easy, it means you've either been practicing it or you are doing it incorrectly. You must also keep your rib cage and shoulders in contact with the ground, so that you definitely feel a good pull on the waist.

Now do it again, this time breathing in as you stretch to the position in Figure 6.8, out as you return to the position in Figure 6.7.

Once you have coordinated this, start again and use the right leg.

Figure 6.7

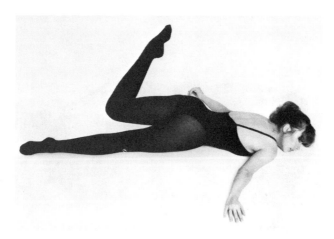

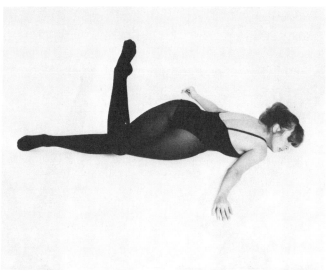

Figure 6.8

PYGMALION (PIG-MAY-LEE-ON): This exercise shapes the whole leg, the buttocks, and the abdomen, but most work is done in shaping the thighs.

Lie on your back, and lift yourself to the position in Figure 6.9.

Point your toes, legs together, and support yourself strongly on the hip bone with your hands as shown.

Breathe freely, while performing circles with each leg, first clockwise and then counterclockwise.

You can see in Figure 6.10 that the legs must go wide apart.

The more vertically the legs are placed, the more work is done on the abdomen.

PHEME (FEE-ME): This exercise can help lift the bust but there it is also a good exercise for the shoulders and arms. The main shaping effect is on the contour of the join of the hip to the body.

Lie on your back and raise your legs as shown in Figure 6.11. Press your palms against your knees. Take a deep breath and press hard against your knees, pressing back with your legs. Hold for a count

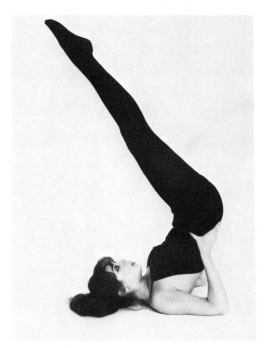

Figure 6.9

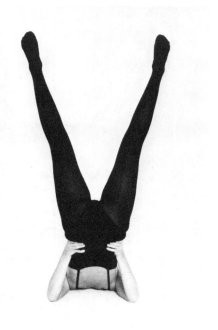

Figure 6.10

Figure 6.11

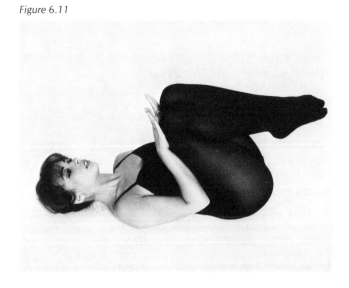

of five, and then exhale through a count of ten as you decrease the pressure. Now, breathe in again through a count of ten as you gradually increase the pressure. Hold as before, and exhale with reduced hand pressure.

Get into a rhythm and work hard with this excellent shaper of the groin and thigh.

ROUTINE MASSAGE

Your body can respond to the shaping movements of your hands almost like a sculptor shapes clay. The secret is to follow the natural contours of the tissues, thereby consolidating the work you have done exercising the muscles.

Routine massage increases blood flow to the skin and fat layer beneath, thereby aiding fat loss when your calorie intake is correct. I have found some women, although they lose fat on slimming diets, still retain localized pockets of fat, especially on the thighs and belly. In studio work, we always use some massage for these people, and you can do a lot using the following sequences.

Practice them with a little oil or cream for lubrication, but once you know the routine do it regularly in the shower.

Sequences

CONTOURS FROM THIGH OVER HIP TO SIDE OF WAIST Place your hands firmly and flat on your thigh as shown in Figure 6.12. Press and draw them up smoothly to the position in Figure 6.13. Repeat this five times. Then work on the other thigh.

CONTOUR FROM SIDE OF THIGH OVER HIP TO WAIST TO BUST Use one hand firmly on the thigh as in Figure 6.14 and draw it up smoothly to the positions in Figures 6.15 to 6.16. Repeat five times, and then work on the other side of your body.

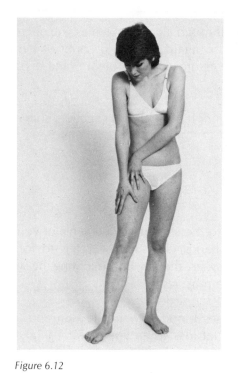

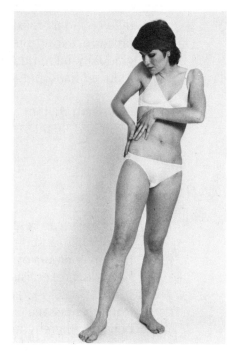

Figure 6.12

Figure 6.13

Figure 6.14

Figure 6.15

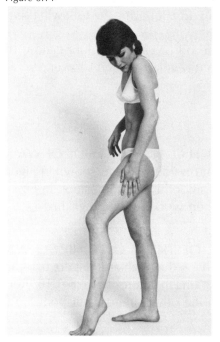

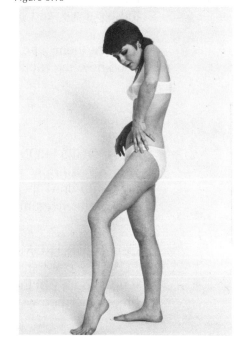

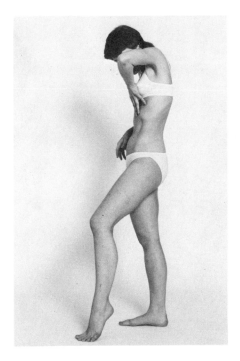

Figure 6.16

CONTOUR FROM BACK OF THIGH OVER BUTTOCKS TO SMALL OF THE BACK Starting just below the knee, move the shin up in smooth strokes with the flat of your hand. Repeat 10 times, and then work on the other leg with your other hand.

CONTOURS FROM INSIDE CALF UP TO SIDE OF BELLY This contour is crucial for a strong and good-looking body, and should be done regularly every time you take a shower. At first do it slowly, feeling for your own natural lines on the muscles and ligaments. Start at the position in Figure 6.17. Note how the first two fingers are pressed firmly into the skin. Draw the hands up along the inside of the thigh as in Figure 6.18, up to the crotch as in Figure 6.19, and then more gently, follow the line on each side of the pubic hair to the position in Figure 6.20. From the position in Figure 6.20 go straight up to the position in Figure 6.21.

Take your hands off your body, and start all over again. Do this 10 times. When you become adept, use the flat of the hand as well for even firmer work.

You can increase the efficiency of this sequence further by cupping

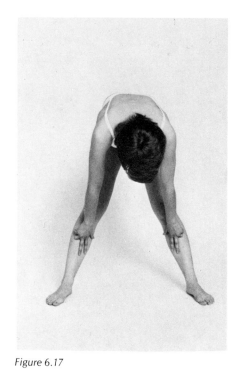

Figure 6.17

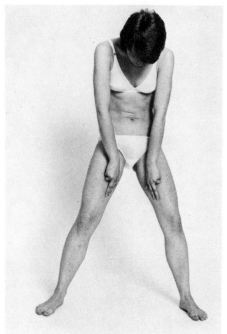

Figure 6.18

Figure 6.19

Figure 6.20

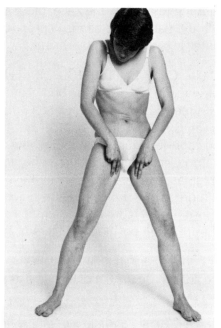

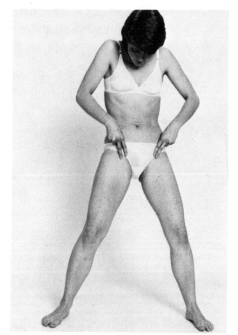

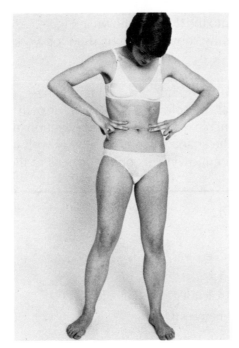

Figure 6.21

Figure 6.22

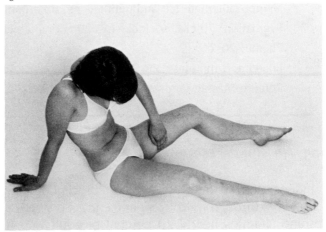

the hand deep into the thigh as shown in Figure 6.22 when a sitting position (not for the shower!) can be used for work on one leg at a time.

The idea behind this sequence is to familiarize yourself with the distribution of fat, muscle, and bone in your own body. For stubborn fat areas, increase the massage in repetition and effort. When drying, follow the shape of your own body with the towel, using upward sweeping movements on the legs as in the massage.

PROTOCOL

Athena: 5 x

Callisto: 1 x very very slowly

Cassandra: 5 x

Nymph: 10 x left leg, 10 x right leg

Phaedra: 2 minutes (Day 2)

Athena: 10 x

Cassandra: 10 x

Athena: 5 x

Nymph: alternate left and right legs, to do a minimum of 20

Pygmalion: 20 circles clockwise, 20 counterclockwise

Pheme: 20 x

Phaedra: 3 minutes (Day 2)

Routine Massage: in shower

ADEQUATE NUTRITION

Independent surveys reveal that 10 percent of Western women are anaemic through mild iron deficiency. Surveys also show that for some vitamins nearly 20 percent of adults are mildly deficient. This level of deficiency depresses vitality and looks, usually through your skin. Clearly, to make progress in this program your diet must provide adequate levels of minerals and vitamins.

A lack of vitamins eventually leads to serious diseases, but long before such illnesses occur minor deficiencies depress vitality and impair looks. Here is how and why.

The majority of vitamins are destroyed by the high temperature processing of food, one of the reasons why freshness is so important to your diet.

VITAMIN A This vitamin is found only in foods of animal origin, but it can be made from the red pigment beta carotene found in red and yellow vegetables. Liver is a particularly rich source of vitamin A. Vitamin A is essential for healthy eyes and clear skin. You need 750 units a day. See the table in Day 7 for natural sources.

VITAMIN D The sun's rays act on animal fats and fungi fats in your skin to produce vitamin D. The only good sources of preformed vitamin D are fish liver oils, such as cod liver oil. Vitamin D is essential for a strong skeleton. Adults eating a varied diet who maintain an outdoor life obtain adequate levels of this vitamin.

VITAMIN K Plant foods, especially dark green vegetable leaves such as sprouts, are good sources of this vitamin, which is essential for healthy blood.

VITAMIN E Adults require 25 mg a day of vitamin E, a level not reached by most Western diets, but achieved when on a diet containing whole wheat cereals and bread, along with fresh fruits and eggs.

Vitamin E reduces internal damage done by natural waste products in the tissues.

VITAMIN C Adults require at least 60 mg a day of vitamin C or ascorbic acid, about the amount in two fresh oranges. Twice this level is easily achieved on a fresh mixed diet and saturates the blood and tissues. It is essential for healthy skin.

VITAMIN B_1, THIAMINE Mild thiamine deficiency results in loss of appetite, anxiety, irritability, and lack of energy. Skin health also suffers. Women require 2 mg of thiamine daily. Whole grains, liver, and yeast are all good sources.

VITAMIN B_2, RIBOFLAVINE Good sources of vitamin B_2 are egg yolks and whole grain cereals. Dairy produce is an important source because of milk. Mild riboflavine deficiency produces lassitude and deterioration of skin. Women require 1.3 mg daily.

VITAMIN B_3, NICOTINIC ACID, NIACIN, NICOTINAMIDE Mild deficiency reduces vigor and skin health. Women require 15 mg of nicotinic acid each day. Good sources are liver, egg yolks, and whole grain cereals.

VITAMIN B_{12} Without B_{12}, severe anaemia develops. This vitamin is not found in plants but meats and dairy products. Unlike most vitamins, vitamin B_{12} can be stored in the liver. Several months supply can be stored in healthy human livers.

FOLIC ACID This acid is found in fresh green vegetables and liver. Deficiency leads to anaemia. Approximately .4 mg are required daily.

VITAMIN B, PYRODOXINE Deficiency of this vitamin depresses vigour and skin health. Meat and the bran of cereals are good sources.

PANTOTHENIC ACID This acid is found in most foods but the best sources are eggs, fresh vegetables, liver, and yeast. It is essential for healthy skin.

BIOTIN This vitamin is particularly important for general health. While yeasts and bacteria make biotin, we obtain most of our biotin from the bacteria living in our intestines.

Day 7

BUST

Women with small breasts can go without a bra at any time, even when manually working hard, running, or engaged in any sport no matter how strenuous.

Larger breasts will, however, move about uncomfortably when the elasticity of the skin, the fluid pressure, and the supportive tissues inside the breasts are unequal due to sudden strains. This leads to a tearing of the tissues, which may or may not be painful.

Brassieres are, therefore, useful at certain times. Note that good bras:

Have no heavy metal catches,
Do not cover all of the breast,
Are made of thin, attractive, material with pores, to let the skin breathe.

YOU DON'T NEED BRAS:

In bed,

At home,

On warm days (put a little talc under your breasts if they are large),

Swimming,

When making love,

When eating,

When relaxing on the beach,

When watching TV, films, plays.

IO (EE-OH): Io lifts the bust from the inside top.

Assume the position as shown in Figure 7.1. Put your foot against the inside of your thigh. Clasp your hands, breathing in. Pull tightly on your hands while pulling in your tummy as in Figure 7.2. Hold for 15 seconds and exhale. Relax and switch your leg position and repeat.

Note how defined the waist becomes (Figure 7.2). The purpose of the leg position is to emphasize work on one side of your waist, and as you cross over, the other.

Figure 7.1

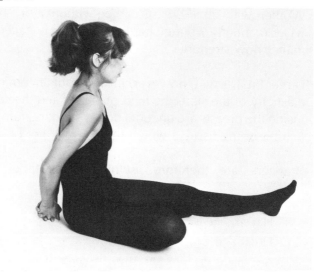

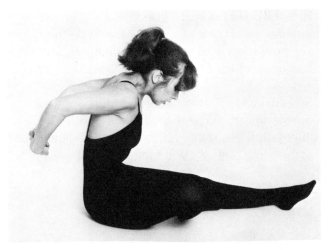

Figure 7.2

<u>HERA (HE-RAH)</u>: Hera allows the breast to hang entirely free while the large muscles on the side of the chest are strengthened. The result is a firming of the bust's foundation.

Assume the position in Figure 7.3, with your legs about 18 inches apart. Breathe in and pull on your legs as you pull your tummy in. Hold for 15 seconds, exhale. *Caution:* Do this gently at first.

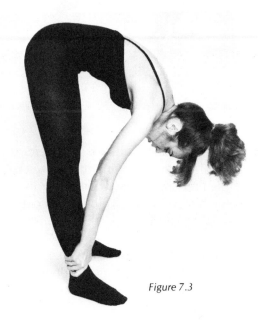

Figure 7.3

PHOEBE (FEE-BEE): Phoebe is an exercise for the bust foundation muscles. Look in a mirror as you do this exercise and you will see how the breasts are lifted when you press. Phoebe is used in conjunction with the following exercise, Lamia.

Sit as in Figure 7.4 and note how the hands are placed palms down on the knees. As you breathe in gently, gradually press on the knees until you attain full pressure, pressing back with your knees at the same time. As you breathe out, gradually relax the pressure.

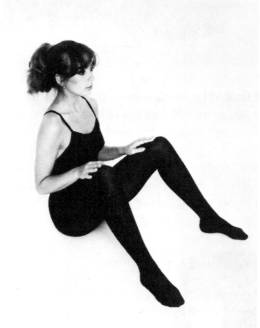

Figure 7.4

LAMIA (LAY-MEE-AH): Lamia is an exercise for the abdomen and bust as well as strengthening the back. Like Phoebe, it exercises the arms and shoulders while using the hands in a power position, something they can well do with considering how many gadgets have taken our hand function from us.

Assume the position as shown in Figure 7.5. Note how the hands strongly grip the legs, about 3 inches down from the knee.

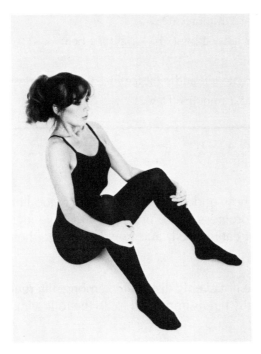

Figure 7.5

As you breathe in, pull on the legs with increasing strength, so that when you have completely inhaled, you are pulling with maximum strength. Now push the air out as you gradually relax the pull on your legs.

Repeat from beginning, but this time pull the abdomen in as you breathe in, and let it relax as you breathe out.

Now try it again, and add this further refinement. As you breathe in, sit as tall as you can on your buttocks, and relax them as you breathe out.

PROTOCOL

Phoebe: 10 x

Lamia: 10 x

Io: 5 x left leg bent, 5 x right leg bent

Hera: 10 x

Phaedra: 2 minutes (Day 2)

Io: 10 x left leg bent, 10 x right leg bent

Hera: 5x

Io: alternate left and right leg for 20 repetitions of the exercise.

Phaedra: 2 minutes (Day 2)

HOW TO EAT WELL

You should now understand that only with good nutrition can you expect real progress in the program. We have identified the main principles of eating well, and now will refine these ideas even in more detail.

Nutrients are not evenly distributed among different foods, so to be sure your daily fare is improved, scan the following nutrient source analyses.

VITAMIN A activity is high in fish livers, vitaminized margarine, liver, and red palm oil. While dairy produce and red and yellow vegetables provide good amounts too.

VITAMIN D activity is high in cod liver oil, and halibut liver oil, while herring, salmon, sardines, eggs (whole and yolk), and butter are average but useful sources. Dairy products and meat, although low in vitamin D, are important because they are staple foods in our diets.

VITAMIN B, B_1; THIAMINE, activity is high in yeast, bran, whole wheat, and brown rice, while fruits and vegetables, pork, beef, mutton, fish, milk, and eggs are very useful sources.

VITAMIN C activity is high in black currants, rose hips, and all citrus fruits, while fruits and green leafy vegetables are important sources too.

VITAMIN B_2, RIBOFLAVIN activity is high in wheat, wheat bran, wheat germ, barley, fish, beef, mutton, pork, liver, kidney, eggs, cheese, cocoa, chocolate, brewer's yeast, yeast extract, wheat germ extracts, and meat extracts, while corn, oatmeal, wheat flour, cashew nuts, green leafy vegetables, fruit, milk, and beer are useful sources too.

VITAMIN B_3, NIACIN activity is high in wheat bran, wheat germ meal, rice, sorghum, wheat flour, fish, beef, mutton, pork, liver, kidney, brewer's yeast, and meat extract, while corn, oatmeal, rice, wheat flour, cashew nuts, fruit, cocoa powder, and chocolate are important sources too.

IRON activity is high in red meat and fish, while eggs, nuts, cereals, and green leafy vegetables are important.

CALCIUM activity is high in cheese, milk, nuts, pulses, roots, squashes, and stem vegetables, while eggs, cereals, and fruits, are important sources too. Small fish, eaten whole, such as sardines, are also high sources.

During the program write down what you eat, and then check to see if you have included high sources of these nutrients in your daily food intake. If you note that some nutrients are constantly being left out in the high source category, make sure that next day you include a high source for that nutrient in some of your meals. Note that vitamin D is mostly made from other substances when your skin is exposed to sunlight. There is no need to bake yourself because the effect of sunlight on the face during outdoor work or play is usually sufficient, although bare legs are even more effective. The foods important in providing these nutrients for vitamin D synthesis can be found in meat, dairy products, and fungi (mushrooms). Consequently, there is no need to eat fish oils.

Cooking

Having identified the good foods, you must now keep your meals varied and apply the following hints to cooking.

SCRAMBLED EGGS Prepare as before but don't use butter. Use a nonstick pan instead.

CASSEROLES AND STEWS Use traditional recipes, but meticulously cut off the fat from the meat. Don't use white flour, substitute brown rice as a thickener instead. Add ice cubes to gravies because fat will collect around them. Discard the fat and ice cubes.

PASTRIES AND FRUIT CAKES Get a large salt shaker and fill it with brewer's yeast. Get into the habit of sprinkling it on soups (a little, it is bitter) and cereals. Experiment with traditional recipes by reducing sugar, and use more fruit. Use whole meal flour, not white.

MEAT AND FISH You can keep meat moist when grilling by using onions, which you then discard.

SALADS Your salads should be as varied as possible, with lettuce, fruits, nuts, radishes, cucumbers, peppers, cabbage, celery, carrots, and so on. Fruit salads should also be varied and mixed.

New Kinds of Meals
Mix fruits with cereals. Cereals (oats, shredded wheat, brown rice, bran, wheat germ) mixed with banana, apples, oranges, tangerines, and melon are just a few. Dried fruits are also available in large variety, such as raisins, currants, and dates. Yogurt that is natural, not sweetened, can also be a treat. Unfortunately, most commercial yogurts contain sugar, but you can make up your own. Get in the habit of using these dishes for two meals of the day. Other snack ideas for one person follow.

POACHED EGGS Bring water to boil, add ½ teaspoon of vinegar, break egg into it. Leave two minutes gently boiling. Eat with wholemeal toast.

SARDINES ON TOAST Open and empty a small can of sardines onto strong tissue paper to absorb the excess oil. Grill wholemeal bread on one side, turn, half toast and add fish. Add black pepper to taste. This is delicious with sliced tomatoes, or a squeeze of lemon.

KIDNEYS Grill 2 to 4 ounces of kidneys, prepare toast as above.

BACON AND TOMATOES Grill 1 to 3 slices of unsmoked bacon. Cut tomatoes in half; grill. Serve with toast.

HERB OMELETTE Break an egg into a cup, whisk with mixed herbs, add to pan containing ½ to 1 teaspoon of vegetable oil (sunflower, safflower, olive). Turn once.

Soups
Using any good cookbook, follow the recipes for soup but leave out the fat, sugar, and white flour ingredients. Here are some new recipes for experimenting.

TOMATO You will need one cup of vegetable water (from boiling potatoes, cabbage, and so on) and two to three medium-sized tomatoes.

Drop the tomatoes into boiling water, then remove and peel the skin. Combine tomatoes and vegetable water in blender. Pepper, herbs may be added to taste. Gently heat. Serves 1 to 2 people.

VEGETABLE SOUP Combine 4 to 6 ounces of any single vegetable, or mixed vegetable, for example two leaves of cabbage and ¼ cup of small peas. Boil then combine in blender. Add herbs to taste and heat. Serves 1 to 2 people.

Main Dishes
Veal, steak, fish, and pork, will all grill very easily. Remove the excess fat and grill on foil. Keep meat moist with onion (to discard). Herbs can be added if you wish. I like rosemary on river trout and parsley on veal. Serve with one or more boiled vegetables. Try trout with small fresh new potatoes and sliced carrots.

CHOPS Cut the fat and bone away after grilling but before serving.

CHICKEN Grilled or roasted chicken smells good, tastes good, and feels good. The bones are hard and the gristle tough. A broiled or fried chicken smells bad, feels bad, tastes bad, and its bones are soft. Grill, roast your chicken.

FISH Fish is a wonderful main meal (as well as a starter) and can be deliciously grilled, poached, or baked in foil packed with herbs and a drop of wine to keep it moist. Many varieties are freely available; cod, whitebait, plaice, salmon.

PASTAS Excellent, if you use whole-grain pastas.

SWEETS AND DESSERTS There are so many hundreds of fruits, that dessert can always be a surprise. You can eat fruit raw, boiled, baked, with yogurt, and with a wholemeal biscuit. Fruit is a never-ending source of refreshment and pleasure.

CHEESE There are many hundreds of cheeses. They make good snacks with fruit.

WINES A glass of wine gives pleasure and helps digestion. Dry wines are preferable for slimming.

Day 8

ARM AND BREAST SHAPING

One woman in two takes a B-cup bra. While larger and smaller sizes are evenly distributed, there are as many women with A-cup breasts as those with C cup and larger.

In all women, the shape of the breast depends on skin elasticity, fluid pressure, and the muscles underneath the breasts.

During sexual excitement, the breast size can increase by half again. Women with fulfilling lives tend to have firmer breasts because the fluid pressure is maintained. A sense of pleasure in the body, not merely from sex, increases this pressure. In very healthy women, a steady pulse of lymph and blood can easily be felt flowing into the breast to maintain its contour.

Very few women have identical breasts, there being a good 10 percent difference in volume, with the right one being larger than the left, for right-handed women.

During menstruation the breasts swell. A difference of up to 3 inches in bust measurement can occur.

These are the facts you have to work with during the program. *Pleasure* is used for contour, *exercise* to increase blood flow, and *strong hard work* is used to strengthen the muscles beneath the breasts.

However there are some regular routines to carry out:

When in the shower always cup the breasts and press with your hands upwards, raising the breasts. Then let go, and start again. This usually results in the nipple swelling, so that fatty secretions are not trapped in the puckered skin. The massage also improves blood circulation, and lymph supply too.

If you find during sex that you have little feeling in your breasts, it means you have the cut-off breast feeling syndrome, which is common.

Kissing, licking, fondling, stroking, and massaging all excite the breasts, so that blood pumps in very strongly. In healthy women, the blood flow is so strong you can actually see the breasts rise, and the bust takes on the form of firmness and good contour it basically has. Through inept sex, many women have given up this part of their bodies, and the blood flow does not occur, resulting in cold and nonparticipating breasts. This is a most unhealthy state because just as the lips of the vagina swell and become hot, so should the nipple and breasts.

I am trying to emphasize that just as in healthy women there is a good flow to the vagina at all times, there should also be to the breasts. These flows are as natural as breathing, and when they cease it implies tenseness, anxiety, or sheer unhappiness, while the good flow and warmth reveals health.

Consequently, to develop healthy breasts, you need more than mere exercises that actuate the chest muscles—you need the pleasure flow exercises. I have included them in the Protocol section.

HARMONIA (HAR-MOE-KNEE-AH): Assume the position in Figure 8.1, and note how the feet are symmetrically placed, the toes not curled. The back is straight as well.

Place your fingertips together as shown. Breathe in slowly as you increase the pressure on your fingertips by pressing hard.

When you have completely inhaled, hold for a count of five with maximum pressing, and then exhale slowly as you gradually release the pressure on your fingertips.

As you get better at this exercise, take 15 seconds to exhale as you gradually relax pressure.

Do this in front of a mirror and you will see how the breast is lifted.

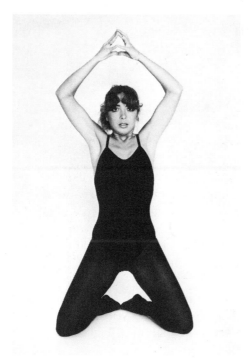

Figure 8.1

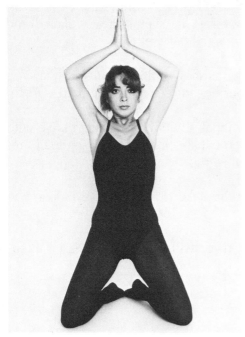

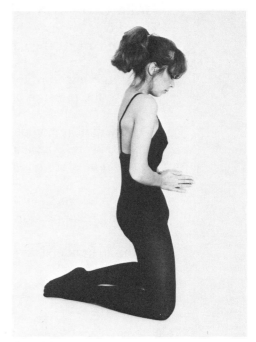

Figure 8.2   Figure 8.3

DAPHNE (DAF-KNEE): This exercise is similar to Harmonia and performed exactly in the same way, although this time just the palms of the hands are together, not the fingertips. (See Figure 8.2.) The effect is to lift the bust, just as with Harmonia, but the breasts are brought closer together. Also the work is very much harder. Accordingly, Harmonia is the warm up, and Daphne is the hard, power exercise for tissue work.

CIRCE (SER-SEE): This is a very hard exercise, so do it gently at first and build up the pressure.

Start at the position in Figure 8.2, as in Daphne. Breathe in, and press as hard as you can as you sweep in a gentle arc while exhaling to reach the position in Figure 8.3.

Relax the hands, then press hard and inhale as you sweep up to the position in Figure 8.2 again, still keeping the pressure on the hands. Exhale as you come down again. When you are doing this well, you will take 10 seconds to breathe in, and breathe out.

Do this exercise in front of a mirror and you will see that you are working on the belly muscles as well, while lifting the breasts.

PROTOCOL

Harmonia: 10 x ⎫
Daphne: 10 x   ⎬   Slowly and with strong pressure
Circe: 10 x   ⎭

Phaedra: 2 minutes (Day 2)

Harmonia: 10 x ⎫
Daphne: 10 x   ⎬   Quickly with little pressure
Circe: 10 x   ⎭

Venus: 3 x (Day 5)

Harmonia: 1 x ⎫   With *maximum pressure* and a breathing
Daphne: 1 x   ⎬   cycle of 15 seconds in, 15 seconds out
Circe 1 x   ⎭

Phaedra: 3 minutes (Day 2).

Day 9

Massage is an important beauty and health aid because it increases circulation and corrects the natural sag of tissue by stimulating the muscles underneath the skin.

You can follow this massage sequence best during a shower, when the water provides a natural lubricant. Learn the first sequences in front of a mirror, using a little moisturizing cream.

The lines of massage follow the natural contours along the bones and muscles. Note that almost all the movements are upwards and outwards, helping to teach the muscles to lift, not sag.

Massage Sequences

General Instructions
Make sure *only your fingertips touch* the skin, not your nails. Look at the figures carefully. Once you reach the end position of the massage movement, *take your fingertips off your face and start*

again. The sequence takes about five minutes to do properly. It is a good idea to use the relaxing methods you have already learned, then begin the massage.

RELAXATION SEQUENCE: Look into the mirror, say ''Cheese'' three times, and then give a really good smile, which activates many muscles. Hold the smile for a count of three, relax, and repeat three more times.

An entirely different set of muscles is used for pouting. Begin in the relaxed state as shown in Figure 9.1, and pout as in Figure 9.2 (hold for count of five) three times.

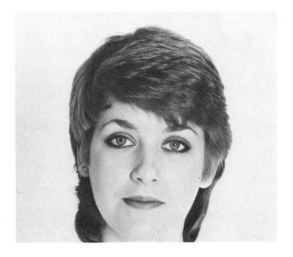

Figure 9.1

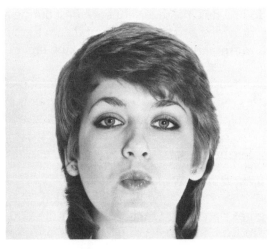

Figure 9.2

BRIDGE OF THE NOSE SEQUENCE: Begin as shown in Figure 9.3, making sure your fingertips, not your nails are in contact with your skin. Apply slight steady pressure, and pull your hands steadily out to your temples in a very flat U curve. Repeat 10 times.

Next, start higher up, as shown in Figure 9.4, and sweep out to the temple as before in a low U curve. Figure 9.5 shows the halfway stage. Repeat 10 times.

Now use the tips of your fingers on the forehead as shown in Figure 9.6, sweeping out as before. Repeat five times.

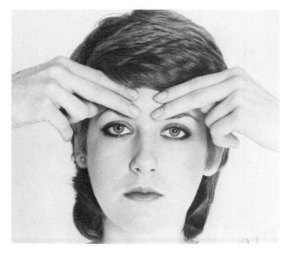

Figure 9.3

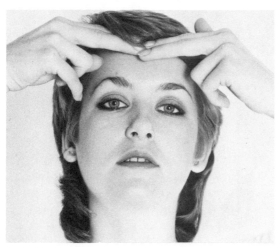

Figure 9.4

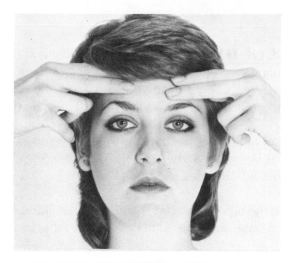

Figure 9.5

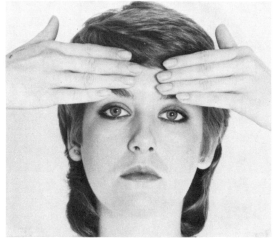

Figure 9.6

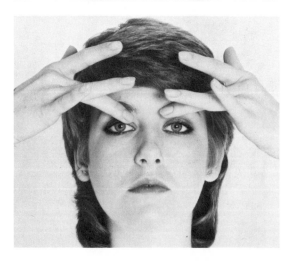

Figure 9.7

84

EYEBROW SEQUENCE: Apply your middle finger as shown in Figure 9.7 under your eyebrow. Apply steady pressure and sweep in an upward curve along the eyebrow. Repeat five times.

EYE SEQUENCE: Be delicate and gentle in this sequence. Do not drag your skin and stay on your cheekbone, not on the soft skin beneath the eye.

Begin the massage at the inside of your eye as shown in Figure 9.8 and sweep very gently and slowly ending as in Figure 9.9. Only your middle finger is in contact. Repeat five times.

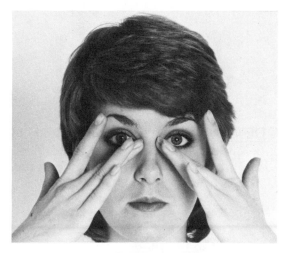

Figure 9.8

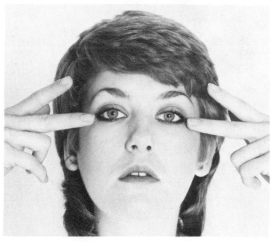

Figure 9.9

CHEEK SEQUENCE: Apply pressure with the first and second fingers, by the tips alone. Start from the position in Figure 9.10. With a U curve, move to the bottom of the ears. Repeat seven times.

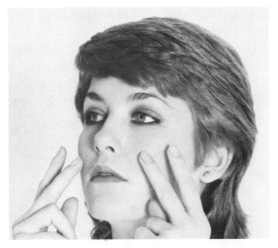

Figure 9.10

LIP SEQUENCE: With the tip of your second finger, apply pressure just below your nose but above your upper lip as in Figure 9.11. Sweep in a shallow curve to the top of the ear. Repeat 10 times.

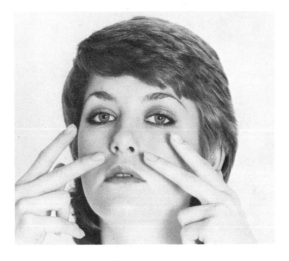

Figure 9.11

NECK SEQUENCE: Use the backs of your fingers to massage yourself under your chin as in Figure 9.12. First use your left hand and then your right hand. Keep firmly in contact with your neck until you reach your chin, then break off and start again. Don't touch your Adam's apple! Do this for a total of 30 seconds.

Place the tips of your first and second fingers at the sides of your neck. Start at about the level of your Adam's apple. Slide your fingers straight up as in Figure 9.13 to reach the jaw line, then follow the jaw back to your ears. Break off, and repeat 16 times in all.

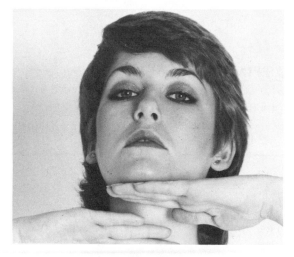

Figure 9.12

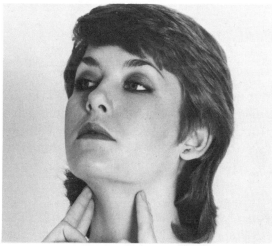

Figure 9.13

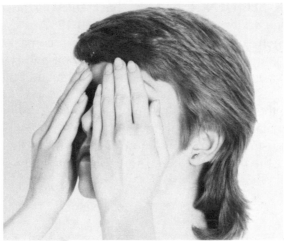

Figure 9.14

EYE CUPPING: Rest your eyes by covering them gently and firmly with cupped hands as shown in Figure 9.14. Sit in a dark or dull room (not in the shower). Open your eyes. Stare into the blackness as you feel the tiredness leaving your eyes.

PROTOCOL

Facial Massage

Repeat Protocol for Day 6, adding 6 repetitions of Venus (Day 5).

ROUTINE HEALTH CARE OF THE FACE

Teeth

Brush your gums rather than your teeth to keep blood circulation going. Brush up from the gum. Use toothpicks after each meal to remove food particles. Keep teeth clean with toothpaste and a toothbrush. Have dental check every six months.

Eyes

Shield your eyes against draught, dust, and excessive sun. Use sunglasses that cut out ultraviolet light. If you squint or frown, see an optician.

Hair

Shampoo your hair as little as you can. It is much better to take longer with less shampoo using a hand massage and running warm water. Remember that dyeing—not tinting or rinsing—can damage the hair's surface. Dry hair with mild hot air, as too much heat splits hair. Get a healthy sheen by brushing with a close-bristled brush over the hair's surface. Invigorate the hair roots by brushing with a large-bristled brush. Never use a wire brush. Invest in a very large-toothed blunt comb for routine combing every day. Spend money on the cut of your hair, not perming, curling, or dyeing. Because hair style depends on the cut, this expertise is expensive.

Day 10

THIGHS AND BACK

PANDORA (PAN-DOOR-AH): Pandora is a particularly beautiful exercise and one that works the whole body. It is particularly good at shaping the line from the knee up along the thigh, across the groin to the navel. It also helps pinch in the waist at each side, straightens the lower back and shapes the abdomen.

Pandora is a stretch-contraction exercise where rhythm is gradually built up. There is a considerable workload to it because of the whiplash of the thigh from a lower to a higher position involving the movement of about 30 pounds weight.

Consequently, once you have coordinated the movement, you increase your workload by speeding up the movement, while still retaining rhythm and grace, and eventually putting a premium on the oxygen supply.

Pandora is also a first-class aerobic exercise, but unlike jogging because it is a stretching and shaping exercise, not merely an aerating exercise.

Take your position on all fours, knees bent, and thread your left leg to take up the position in Figure 10.1. Stretch the leg as far as it will go, and then draw it out in a graceful curve to reach position as shown in Figure 10.2. Stretch the hip as you reach the top.

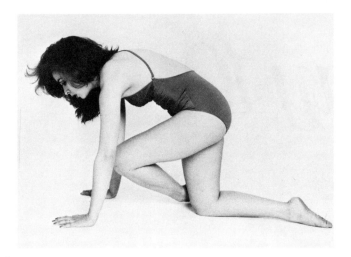

Figure 10.1

Figure 10.2

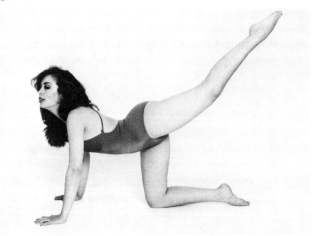

Now bring the leg down and thread it through again as in Figure 10.1, and then withdraw to the position in Figure 10.2 again.

Continue this until you are doing the movement without brushing the floor with the knee or foot of the moving leg.

Once you have reached this stage, work with your right leg.

After completing the workout with the right leg, alternate the legs, breathing in as you thread the leg, out as you raise the leg as shown in Figure 10.2.

Concentrate on rhythm, doing it slowly at first until you have perfected it. An excellent performance is 20 in 20 seconds.

PROTOCOL

Pandora: 20 x

Phaedra: 3 minutes

Pandora: 20 x

Phaedra: x 3 minutes

Pandora: 20 x

Protocol Day 8

Day 11

RHEA (REE-AH): Rhea is a back relaxer. Your back was designed not for standing, but for being on all fours. Consequently, good figure development needs to rest on a well-toned back. For this the back has to be rested. By bending the back in the opposite direction it normally takes, flexibility is enhanced.

Kneel and open the knees, making sure the feet are relaxed and the toes are not curled. Place your elbows and forearms on the floor in front of you, and gradually inch them back until they are well between your knees.

In the position, in Figure 11.1 the back is bent and the forehead can rest on the ground. Use a cushion for your forehead if you wish.

Note the complete symmetry of Rhea. In this position, exhale on a count of ten and let the air come in on a count of five. From time to

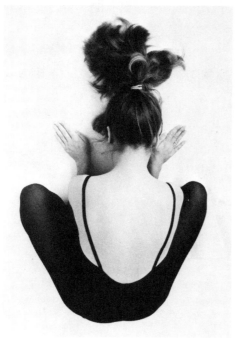

Figure 11.1

time, lift up your back and push your hands forward. Then bring your hands back so the back is bent, while keeping the same rhythm of breathing.

PROTOCOL

Rhea: 3 minutes
Persephone: 7 x (Day 1)
Aphrodite: 7 x (Day 3)
Protocol Day 5

MEDITATION

Daydreaming is one of the most powerful methods of calming and restoring the brain to a quiet, peaceful, well-ordered state. You cannot reach this state by thinking about it, any more than you can get a better body by merely thinking about it. You actually have to do certain things to calm the mind, remove stress, and think and feel more realistically. It is in this practical health-giving way that I use the word "meditation."

Meditation is extremely easy. It is not mystical. It is not even mysterious. The results may be, but the methods are not.

First, the most accessible meditation is by allowing a truth to fix itself in your mind. This process happens all the time. You see a beautiful sky, and the truth of your recognition enters deeply into your mind. Beauty is indeed a meditative tool—you observe beautiful things, feel beautiful things, smell beautiful perfumes, and hear beautiful sounds—all of which calms and enriches your mind. Meditation removes the effects of stress.

Beauty and truth then are reality, but not all truth of course is beautiful, so truth alone is not sufficient for a meditation effect because there must be pleasure in the truth. If you read the following lines you may discover another element of meditation.

> *There is a lot of noise outside of me.*
> *Why should I let that noise come inside of me?*
> *Ships have a compass, a silent guide.*
> *The moon too knows where to go.*
> *The sea has a heart rising and falling,*
> *Even the wind has a path to follow.*
> *I have guidance too,*
> *If I will only listen,*
> *To the whispers in my heart,*
> *They always tell me true.*
> *There is so much noise outside of me,*
> *I have no need for noise inside of me.*

This time there is a calming effect on the mind because the words say something truthful, and say it in such a way that it is reassuringly pleasurable. Part of the pleasure comes from the images, but there is a further element: The words have made a statement that is hopeful. Namely, that you have, we all have, the power to find truth in ourselves without thinking.

You will have noticed by now that I have given my exercises names, and given the pronunciation. You may have found some of the sounds very beautiful and attractive.

If you can remember the most beautiful one *for you,* you have already discovered one of the most powerful techniques of meditation. Because that word, that sound, is the one which will calm your mind most easily and most quickly. We call such a word or sound a *mantra,* and long experience has taught me that each of us have different responses to different sounds at this very deep level. Use the exercise name as *your* mantra. As you go through the program, you will find others.

All you have to do is keep repeating it, audibly if you wish, but eventually in your mind alone, as you work in Rhea *or any other exercise in the program.*

The other important fact is that the more you use a mantra in calmness, deliberation, and with purpose, and the more your body is working harmoniously, the greater the power of the mantra for you. It is a spiritual factor; the more you use it, the more there is of it.

Repeat your mantra, and you will find you begin to think of other things. If they are pleasing, continue, if they are disturbing, then gradually, gently, call back your mantra and repeat it over and over again. When you are feeling refreshed, stop; meditation has done the work we want it to do for you.

These new powers can be used at any time of the day. When anxiety or anger come, use your mantra, and it will free your brain for real, positive thoughts. Then you can deal with the affairs of your life with greater accuracy.

How Far to Go
with Meditation in the Course

In my book *Your Body* (Prentice-Hall, Inc. Englewood Cliffs, N.J., 1982), I describe meditation as a means of entering various gardens and the keys are mantras. The entrance to these gardens are gates, but since there is no actual barrier to us entering, they are gateless gates that really do need a key.

In all there are seven easily identified gardens, each one reached only after going through the one that precedes it. Here we are referring to the first garden, which is entered for pleasure, and the benefits meditation brings.

However, the second garden is for knowledge. Entering this second garden is usually accomplished only after going through a little more trouble, which can be disturbing, though many people enter it without any trouble. This is the reason I say stop the meditation once you have gained refreshment—the sensation is unmistakeable.

If you wish to continue, you may need another mantra in order to pass on from the refreshed state. The average experience goes as follows.

THE FIRST GARDEN

Now you can pick the flowers,
Now you smell their scent.

But if you linger longer
Than it takes to sing a song,
You will find your fancies,
Going where they don't belong.

All you have to do is bear it.
All you have to do is wait.
All you need is patience,
To reach the second gate.

And when it opens and you enter,
You can be there so long,
Time is stitched in ribbons,
And the pattern is so strong.

Here you can remember
All the days gone wrong,
But the knowing makes you better,
And your will more strong.

PASSING FROM THE FIRST
INTO THE SECOND GARDEN

I hear voices, said my friend,
I hear voices in the dark.
I see lights in the shadows,
And cold clutches at my heart.
Now's the time to gamble,
Now's the time for spunk,
You can run if you want to,
But the prize lies out in front.
I must grasp the lightning,
I must make my stand.
Now's the time for fighting,
I have the prize within my hand.

So, if you stop meditation at the stage of refreshment, you are in the first garden. If you continue meditation after this stage, you go into the state I've just described, poised between first and second gardens. For the vast majority of people, it is more profitable to stop at the refreshment stage. Going on is for deeper insights, but you do have to go through the slightly troubling stage I've just described. If you wish to explore your second garden, *wait until you have done the whole 28-day program first.*

On the second use of the program, having become adept at entering the first garden, you can safely enter the second in the following manner. Use the exercise position found most satisfying in the program as your meditative coordinate. Now, choose an entirely different mantra from the one used before. Choose it for its ability to calm without much of a pleasurable sensation. Enter the first garden, *then* use your second mantra.

You will know you have entered the second garden by a much stronger response, wherein you will actually experience your will as a faculty much in the same way as you experienced your new knowledge of your muscles. Stop as soon as you experience the first new insight into your life. Return gently *via your first mantra.*

Day 12

ADVANCED RELAXATION

Polyxena is a pleasure-giving exercise leading to overall improved muscle tone. By this stage of the program, you should easily be able to obtain pleasure from it.

In a class of new students, we find that only one woman in twenty does not reflex into position in Figure 12.1 when the legs are pulled toward the back. The odd one out is always someone who had difficulty in the relaxed breathing, and whose coordination generally is poor marked by a tenseness of the body.

Polyxena is now used by many students to reduce menstrual cramps, and to reduce tensions after a tiring day. It is also a cooling exercise, so that hot flushes can be counteracted to a considerable degree. Like Rhea (Day 11), Polyxena is a major movement for hormonal regulation of the body, inducing deep responses of pleasure, and reducing the effects of stress.

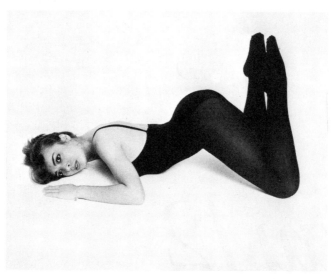

Figure 12.1

Polyxena, Rhea (Day 11), Phaedra (Day 2), and Venus (Day 5) can all be used as regularly in your life as brushing your teeth and cutting your toenails, a basic routine of body strengthening. They can also be used to prevent sexual tension from becoming a discomfort, because if they are regularly practiced, the flow of sensuality throughout the whole body becomes just that, a natural pleasant flow, without sharp, unbalanced tensions. As a result, sexual intercourse becomes more deeply satisfying. Responses occur at a slower, more certain level, rather than sharp peaks of excitement, followed by incomplete satisfaction.

These exercises can also be used by men, where it will be found that tight anal clenching declines, which means that the sensual flow is no longer located in the penis, but travels along the thighs, up the spine, and into the pelvic floor. As a result, erections are more powerful, longer lived, and ejaculations easily controlled. Further, the resultant orgasms are much deeper, not being merely a reflex of the seminal vesicles, but a full response of much more of the body—the thighs, pelvic floor, and large intestines.

A sequence of Rhea, Polyxena, Phaedra, and Venus loosens the unnecessary tensions in the crotch area, so that blood flows more easily. Furthermore, because the muscles relax, the nerves are no longer pinched and can transmit pleasure more favorably. The exercise induces a flooding of the body with endorphins and encephalins, giving pleasure in itself. These changes result in greater quantities of blood perfusing the vagina and vaginal lips. In men, blood volume and pressure, are much increased in the belly and the penis. In both sexes, perfusion is enhanced in the rectum, anus, and colon.

The amount of heat produced is large. This warmth and turgidity is the reason why the exercise Polyxena is cooling. The body heat is located, and the surfaces for radiation of heat away from the body are exposed.

Heat, blood turgidity, and relaxation all mean very satisfying sexuality with particularly long orgasms. Furthermore, these powerful health benefits are obtained without fantasy. One does not have to think sex, as it grows like a flower through the body's energies.

POLYXENA (POL-LEE-ZEE-NA): Lie on your front as shown in Figure 12.2, note the arms and hands are flat on the floor, legs wide, and bent at the knees.

Point your toes.

Inhale, let your back relax, and pull your feet toward your back by bending as much as you can at the knee.

If you are relaxed, you will find your hips rise as shown in Figure 12.1. Press the feet toward the hips strongly and continue to breathe in. Hold for a count of five.

Exhale as you relax your legs back, eventually allowing them to lie on the floor wide apart.

Begin the cycle again by breathing in and bending your legs at the knee until the position in Figure 12.2 is reached again. Hold for a count of five, and then relax as before.

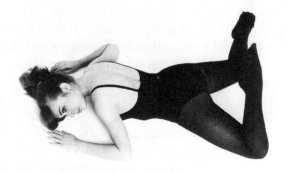

Figure 12.2

When you become adept, you will find this position particularly relaxing, with a pleasurable warmth flowing up the abdomen and spine.

A good cycle is to breathe in and bend the legs over two seconds, hold for three seconds, and then relax down over three seconds.

PROTOCOL

Protocol Day 6
Polyxena: 6 x
Pandora: 20 x (Day 10)
Polyxena: 3 x
Protocol Day 8
Polyxena: 6 x

Day 13

BUTTOCKS

HEBE (HEE-BEE): This exercise is an excellent shaper of the crotch and buttocks, giving tight smooth lines as the excess fat is mobilized.

Sit on the floor as shown in Figure 13.1, and carefully place your legs exactly as shown. Lean back on your hands, so they carry most of the weight.

Now lift your leg, with the foot off the floor, and swing it to your left to the position shown in Figure 13.2.

Once the foot is on the floor, press the leg firmly down and inch it toward your hand as far as you can, thereby stretching the inside of the leg.

When you have gone as far as you can, swing the leg over to the

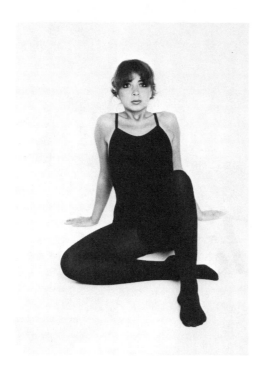

Figure 13.1

Figure 13.2

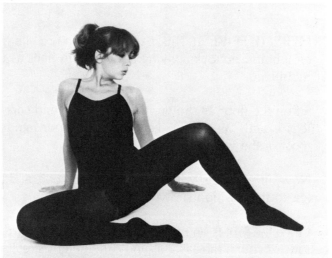

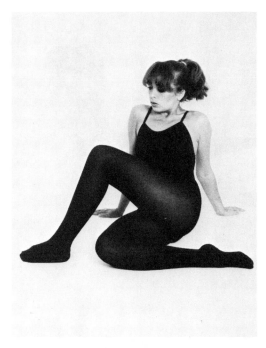

Figure 13.3

position shown in Figure 13.3. Place the foot firmly on the ground, and inch it toward your hand as closely as you can.

Once you have reached the farthest point, thereby stretching the outside of the leg, swing it back to position shown in Figure 13.2.

Repeat this whole sequence until you have the movements coordinated. Exhale during the inching. Inhale when you swing the leg over.

Once you have coordinated the movement of the left leg, change the position so you can now work on the right leg in exactly the same way.

CALLIOPE (KA-LEE-OH-PEE): This is an extremely pretty exercise that stretches the front of the body, thereby leading to tighter lines, particularly on the lines from the hips to the rib-cage and the front of the thighs. As you spread the legs wider, more work is done on shaping the buttocks.

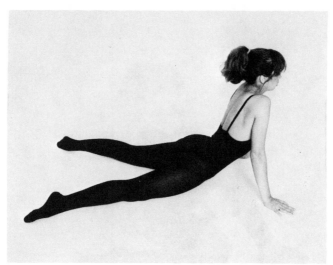

Figure 13.4

Figure 13.5

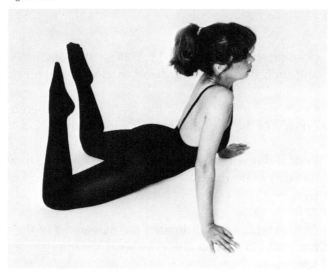

Assume the position shown in Figure 13.4. Note the weight is held by the hands, while the whole of the front of the thigh is lying on the ground. It is essential that the weight be on the thighs and not the knees.

You can inch your way into this by first having your arms bent.

Spread your legs to get maximum weight on the thighs.

Now breathe in on a count of five, as you raise your legs as shown in Figure 13.5, all the time keeping your weight on your thighs. Hold for a count of three, and exhale for a count of ten.

Repeat until you can do this without strain.

PROTOCOL

Hebe: 5 x right, 5 x left
Calliope: 10 x
Phaedra: 2 minutes (Day 2)
Hebe: 10 x right, 10 x left
Calliope: 10 x
Pandora: 30 x (Day 10)
Rhea: 2 minutes (Day 11)
Repeat whole protocol

Day 14

POWER

Controlled power in your body is learning how to increase the muscular tension at will and exploding it into action. Such movements increase the tone of the muscles, thereby improving the general shape of the body.

ISIS (EYE-SIS): Study Figure 14.1 carefully, and you will notice the model has her legs strongly apart, fists clenched, and stands tall and resolute. The tension in the legs comes from putting the weight on the heels and on the outside of the foot where it should be. Assume this position and work at clenching the fists and digging the outside of the foot into the ground, creating tensions all up the body.

DELIA (DEY-LEE-AH): Now study Figure 14.2 just as carefully, and you will see no sign of tension. The weight is evenly distributed on the forward foot and the back foot. The hands are open

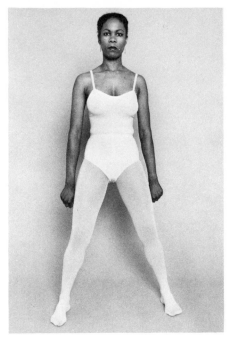

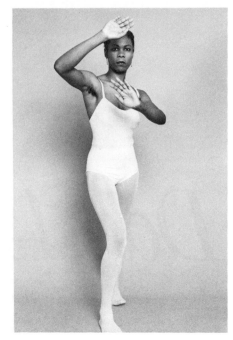

Figure 14.1   Figure 14.2

palmed, resting in position, with no tension other than to hold the position.

Isis is tension, Delia is relaxation from tension. The overall exercise is Isis—Delia, and you do it like this:

Take up a maximum tension Isis, and fill your lungs as you build up the tension in your arms, legs, and torso. When you cannot bear it any more, *explode* into Delia by exhaling through the mouth and stepping fast forward with your right leg, raising your right and left arms to positions in Delia as shown, while at the same time unclenching your fists.

If you have exploded the tension in your body, you will find that you are perfectly relaxed in Delia. It will take time to reach that level of adeptness, but it will teach you so much about the way your body works and help you locate unnecessary tensions in the muscles.

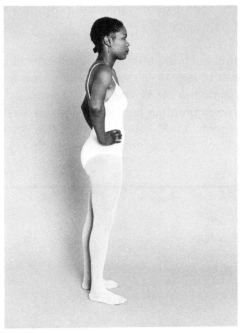

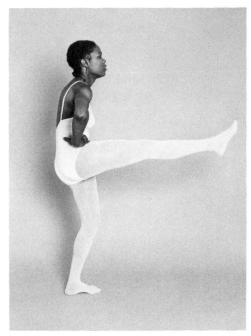

Figure 14.3   Figure 14.4

Stay in Delia for three breath cycles, and then step gently back into Isis, where you build up the tension again, this time exploding with the left leg.

ECHO: Take up position in Figure 14.3, noting the easy, slightly wide leg stance, and hands placed firmly on the hips. Look directly ahead of you, and imagine a point in front of you that you are going to kick. Inhale gently, and then exhale as you bring your right leg up to kick the spot, allowing the leg to only come as high as your hips as in Figure 14.4. Note how the other leg bends a little to cushion the shock. As you bring the leg down again to the position in Figure 14.3, inhale.

Now fix that spot in your mind, so you can aim at it when you next kick. Stand as in Figure 14,3, inhale gently and relaxedly, and then explode into the position in Figure 14.4, kicking with all your force, but cutting the action short as in Figure 14.4, no high kicks! Now relax as you bring the leg back and inhale gently. Reach the position in Figure 14.3 again, then explode into the position in Figure 14.4 again.

Do this several times switching each leg until you have perfected it, and then do it with alternating legs in as quick a succession as you can manage. A good standard of all the relax-tension sequences being performed is one complete leg cycle in half a second, or a cycle of ten movements (L—R—L—R . . .) in five seconds. Remember, it will be some time before you can do this.

PROTOCOL

Isis—Delia: 10 x right, 10 x left

Echo: 10 x, alternate right and left legs

Phaedra: 2 minutes (Day 2)

Isis—Delia: 10 x alternating right and left legs

Phaedra: 2 minutes (Day 2)

Protocol Day 12

Day 15

AEROBIC BODY SHAPING

TERPSICHORE (TURP-SEE-KOR-EE): This is a powerful aerobic exercise, which shapes the waist at the front, and shapes the thigh at front and back.

Stand as shown in Figure 15.1. Place your left leg on ground and raise your right leg. Repeat until you have a rhythm, with the knee at the level of your hips. Now increase the tempo of raising and lowering the legs alternately until you have a rapid free-flowing movement. Continue until tired and/or out of breath. Keep this up until your control of the form of this exercise begins to deteriorate. Immediately go into Phaedra (Day 2) to recuperate. When you have done so, go on now to Hygea.

HYGEA (HI-GEE-AH): Hygea shapes the front of the body.

Take position as shown in Figure 15.2. Note how the feet are placed, and be sure none of your toes are curled. Firmly interleave

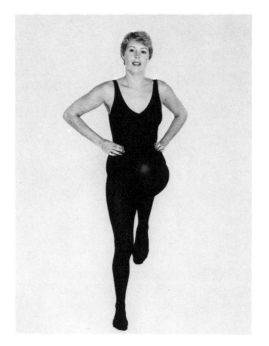

Figure 15.1

Figure 15.2

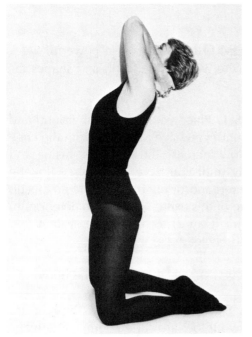

Figure 15.3

your fingers and place them at the back of the neck, but do not press. Inhale deeply as you rise to the position in Figure 15.3, holding your abdomen in as you do so and bringing your arms around so the elbows meet. Hold for a count of three, and then blowing the air out, return to Figure 15.2 and relax. Inhale as you start another cycle.

PROTOCOL

Terpsichore: 3 minutes maximum rate

Phaedra: one minute (Day 2)

Hygea: 10 x

Protocol Days 5, 7 and 8

Repeat this whole sequence once again, finishing with Polyxena (Day 12) before your shower.

Day 16

THIGH AND BELLY SHAPING

Hestia is an exercise that releases relaxant hormones into the bloodstream. The overall body tone is thereby improved and the circulation to the skin enhanced. Hestia can be used as part of the daily relaxant routine to reduce stress. It also soothes the minor back pain many women experience. It is also useful for reducing menstrual cramps.

HESTIA (HESS-TEA-AH): Take the position in Figure 16.1 after working through Phaedra for two minutes (Day 2).

Place the fingertips on the beginning of the arrowed black dots on the thigh as shown in Figure 16.2.

As you inhale, sweep the fingertips up in the direction and along the contour of the arrows, pressing just hard enough with the

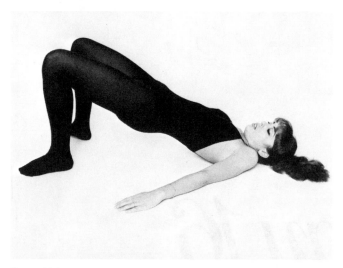

Figure 16.1

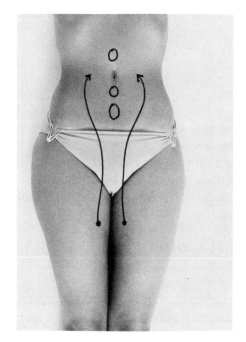

Figure 16.2

fingertips to dig about a quarter of an inch into the skin. Exhale as you reach the arrowheads and lift up the fingers. Transfer the fingers back to the start. Begin again by inhaling.

When you become adept, the upward stroke and the inhalation takes about five seconds, the exhalation also about five seconds.

When you have done seven strokes, put the fingertips of both hands on the first circle area above the navel, and dig with gentle pressure into the skin as you move the fingers in small circles in this area. Breathe gently, exhaling with seven seconds, and inhaling with three seconds.

After 10 breath cycles, move the fingertips to the area indicated by the first circle under the navel, and repeat the fingertip movement and breathing cycles seven times.

Then move on to the lowest circle and repeat the breathing and massaging.

You may find that as you explore this method, you will find an area that is more stimulating, that is it leads to an unmistakeable relaxation of the pelvic floor muscles. Remember it, because this is where you should work in the future.

Finish Hestia off with eleven strokes on the arrow lines as previously described.

PROTOCOL

Hestia plus massage: 3 minutes
Protocol Day 5
Venus: 5 x (Day 5)
Protocol Day 6

Day 17

GROIN SHAPING

Merope is an exercise that stretches the back of the thigh, shapes the bottom and the waist at the side, and improves the line of the crotch and groin.

This is hard effort exercise. As your ligaments and tendons loosen during the program, you may find you need to thrust the hips forward, and bend the back away from the bent leg to get the stretch of Merope.

MEROPE (MERR-O-PEE): Lie on your right side as shown in Figure 17.1. Move about until you are comfortable, taking care with the placement of your legs. You will find your knees are not comfortable when placed exactly on top of one another, which means the left leg is slightly bent at the knee. Make sure too, that your weight is not on your hip bone. Place your left arm on your left hip.

Inhale as you bend your left leg at the knee and bring the thigh up near your chest as shown in Figure 17.2.

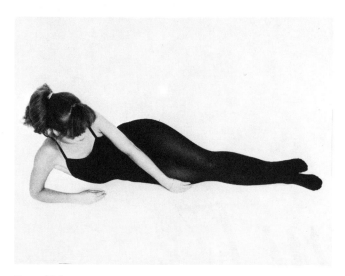

Figure 17.1

Figure 17.2

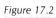

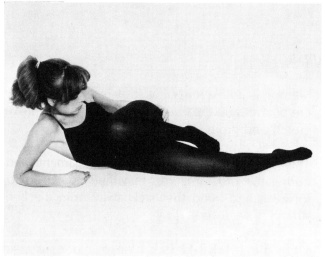

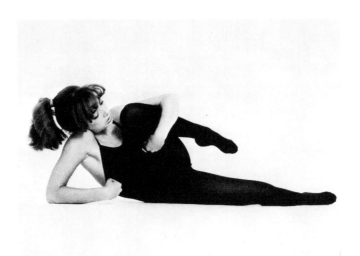

Figure 17.3

Crook your left arm around your knee, and as you fully inhale, pull the leg as close to your chest as you can as shown in Figure 17.3.

Keep pulling hard until you become slightly uncomfortable holding your breath, then let the air out in a whoosh as you slide your leg back to the position in Figure 17.1. Put your arm down to the position in Figure 17.1.

Repeat in a natural rhythm. When adept, the complete movement takes about seven seconds.

Work on your right side until you have coordinated the movements, and then turn to your left side, and repeat, moving your right leg and arm.

PROTOCOL

Merope: 7 x left leg, 7 x right leg
Protocol Day 13
Pandora: 30 x (Day 10)
Protocol Days 7 and 8

Day 18

PENELOPE (PU-NE-LOW-PEE): This exercise is a powerful stretch and control movement that works on the upper back, the waist, and the legs. This exercise is done slowly, with maximum stretch.

Lie on your back as shown in Figure 18.1, legs wide apart, spine relaxed on the floor, and arms a little aside from your body.

Raise your hips about three inches as shown in Figure 18.2, and brace yourself with your arms as you twist your legs to the right as shown in Figure 18.3. Keep your feet in the same position on the floor but raise on your toes if you have the strength.

You should twist far enough to almost touch the ground with your knees, but your hips must not touch the floor. Keep your upper back firmly placed on the ground.

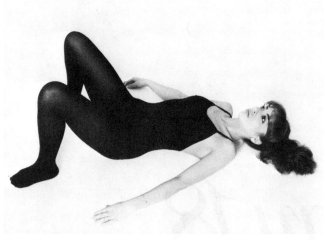

Figure 18.1

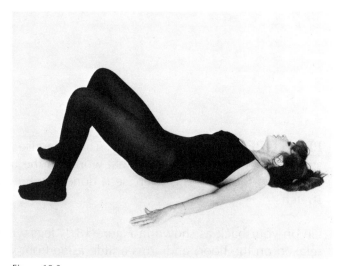

Figure 18.2

Having reached as far as you can go to the right, swing over to the left, as shown in Figure 18.4. Stretch as far as you can go, pressing hard with your hands for balance and purchase.

When you have reached your farthest point, swing over to the other side again as in Figure 18.3. Breathe out as you stretch, breathe in as you swing over.

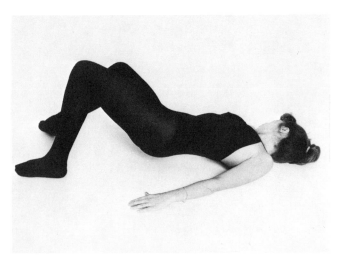

Figure 18.3

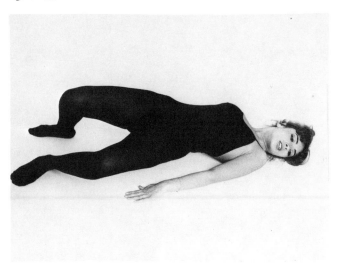

Figure 18.4

PROTOCOL

Penelope: 20 x
Protocol Day 5
Protocol Day 12
Protocol Day 5

Day 19

LEGS

IRENE (EYE-RE-NEE): Irene is a power exercise, sufficiently strong to break down tissue in the thighs, so that it regrows in a stronger and more toned form. It is therefore a shaper of the thighs, particularly in the inside. There is also considerable work done by the abdomen, hence it is a belly and waist shaper.

Experience shows that the majority of women, even when reasonably fit, fail to perform this exercise well. The usual faults are sloppy and too-small circles, no change of pace in movement, bent legs, failure to point the toe, and failure to integrate upper body movement.

All this is the result of failure of determination and concentration. It is impossible to reach your physique potential in shape or fitness without learning and achieving this very fine exercise. It is worth all the sweat and effort you spend exercising the unused muscles of the powerful thighs.

Sit as shown in Figure 19.1. Note the positions of the hands exactly and point the toe of the extended right leg. Now, by pressing on your left leg and hands, raise your hips a little from the floor. Make a large circle slowly with your right leg, moving it up fast and down slow. Begin by moving to the right from the position shown.

As you coordinate this movement well, keep the toe pointed and leg straight. Inhale as you go up, and exhale as the leg comes down. Having perfected this, now circle in the opposite direction.

Having learned Irene for the right leg, change your position so your left leg can be worked. Your right leg becomes your support. Repeat as before.

When really adept, you will find that you raise your hips slightly

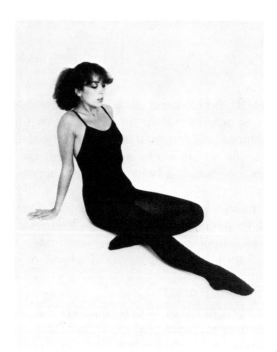

Figure 19.1

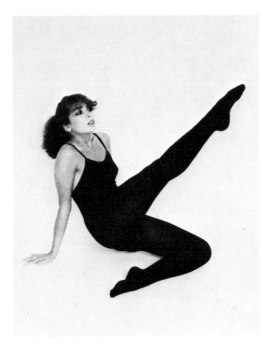

Figure 19.2

higher as you raise the leg. Coming down, your hips will lower but not to the ground as the leg comes down.

It is essential to accelerate speed to the top of the arc, and decelerate slower and slower as you come down from the arc. Also, the toe must be pointed when making a circle. Adept students get the leg well above the head as shown in Figure 19.2. Here the natural back tilt of the head is shown.

PROTOCOL

Irene: left leg 5 x one way, 5 x the other. Repeat with right leg.
Protocol Day 5
Irene: 5 x left leg, each way, 5 x right leg, each way
Protocols Days 6 and 17

Day 20

EXPLOSIVE BREATHING

THETIS (THEE-TEES): In my studio exercise classes, we call this the grunt because it is done so strongly that air is rapidly pushed out of the lungs by the twisting movement, making you grunt. Thetis is a strong, rigid waist-shaper exercise, quite unlike any other in the program.

We have found that one woman in two hundred has a coccyx longer than average, to such an extent it scrapes when sitting. The coccyx is the taillike appendage at the base of the spine, nestling between the buttocks. If you have a coccyx longer than average, do this exercise on a cushion. Everyone, however, should clench their buttocks when sitting on flat hard surfaces to keep the coccyx well away from the ground.

Sit as in Figure 20.1 and spread the legs as wide as possible. Sit tall, with a very straight back and raise the hands well above the

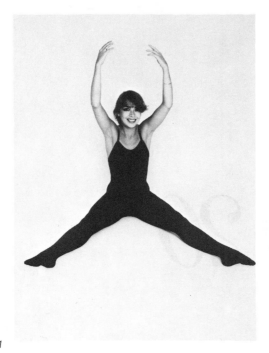

Figure 20.1

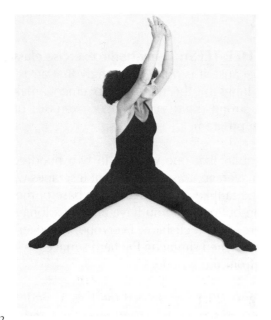

Figure 20.2

shoulders. Now keeping the upper body as rigid as possible, breathe in and gently twist to the left as in Figure 20.2. You will feel air rush out of your mouth, so keep your mouth open. Breathe in and twist to the right, where the same expulsion of air occurs.

Now try the movement with more effort, setting up a rhythm of grunting air out at the twist, then breathing in rapidly as you twist round to the other side, expelling air with the twist.

Having coordinated the movements, you can, clench the fists for greater work impact if your body is strong enough at this stage.

PROTOCOL

Thetis: 2 minutes
Protocol Day 14
Protocol Day 16

Day 21

FULL BODY SHAPING

ATHENE (A-THEENE): Athene is a clearly complex exercise, demanding considerable coordination. The pressing and breathing parts of the cycle lifts the bust, strengthens the arms and wrists, while the ascent from the position in Figure 21.2 gives much work for the back, abdomen, and front of the thighs. The stretching of the body in the squat position improves posture by increasing the flexibility of the tendons and joints, particularly the huge ball-and-socket joint of the thigh. This joint is capable of full circular movements, although it is seldom used as such, except in advanced specialized exercises.

An excellent standard for Athene is 15 in 15 seconds, but it can also be used as a slow exercise wherein the ascent takes a count of 10, and the descent a count of 10, with counts of 10 at the positions in Figures 21.1 and 21.2.

Stand as in Figure 21.1. Note the wide leg stance, the upright

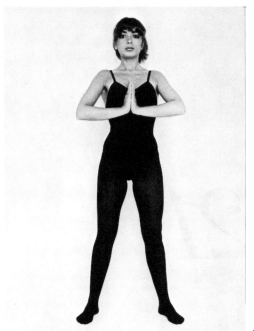

Figure 21.1

Figure 21.2

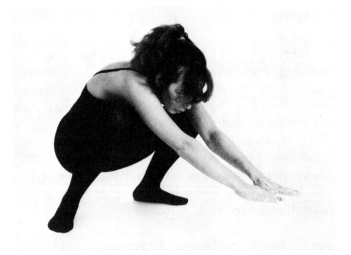

posture, and that the palms of the hands are together, perfectly symmetrical, with the fingertips at about the level of the bust cleavage. Keep your hands and arms away from your body.

Breathe in gently and gradually increase the pressure on your hands by pressing until you are pressing as hard as you can when you finish inhaling. From this position of maximum tension, force the air out as you squat down, pushing your hands away from you as you do so to reach the position shown in Figure 21.2.

Your lungs should now be completely exhaled. Stretch forward as far as you can and widen your knees as far as they will go, so the squat reaches its full expression. Hold for a count of two, and then let the air whoosh in through the mouth as you press hard on your heels to ascend to the position in Figure 21.1 again, pressing your hands as hard as you can while inhaling air. When you are fully pressing and fully inhaled, squat into the position in Figure 21.2 again and breathing out as before.

As you become adept, you may find you need to start with a wider stance. Your weight must be kept on the heels, not the toes.

PROTOCOL

Athene: 5 x slow form
Athene: 10 x fast form
Athene: 10 x slow
Athene: 15 x fast
Protocol Day 17
Protocol Day 7 and 8

Day 22

POWER AND SPEED

Taken together, Ambrosia with its free-flowing movements, and Maia with its graceful control interspersed with violent explosive action, make up an excellent exercise system in themselves. To do them well requires considerable practice and skill.

AMBROSIA (AM-BROSE-EE-AH): Ambrosia is an aerobiotic exercise, which is also a good coordination developer and shaper of the inner thighs.

Stand as in Figure 22.1 and crook the thumbs as shown. Leap and spread the legs, descending to the position in Figure 22.2. Without pausing, leap by pushing up on the toes and balls of the feet to the position in Figure 22.1 again. Continue until a good rhythm is established. Your coordination improves as you leap higher and higher.

On the descent breathe out, and on the ascent, breathe in.

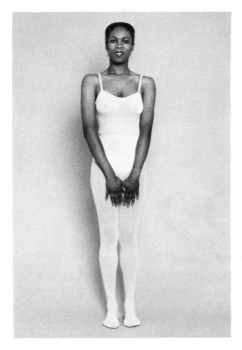

Figure 22.1

Figure 22.2

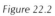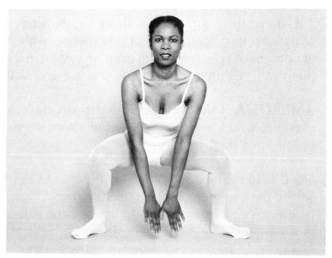

MAIA (MAY-EE-AH): This exercise is another sequence for coordination and rhythmic control but this time not aerobiotic. Deep breathing is not essential. The aim is for graceful, rhythmic movements, with balance so well adjusted that you can stop at any point in perfect equilibrium during the movement.

Study Figure 22.3 carefully. Note that the left leg is forward and the right backward, with weight evenly distributed on each. Now observe the hands. The right hand is held lower than the left hand, but in each case the palm faces away from the body. Imagine you are pushing your palms against the wind.

Still in the position in Figure 22.3, raise the right arm to shoulder level, and the left arm to just above hip level. Remain pushing against the wind. The arms are now in the position in Figure 22.4. Practice the arm movement alone a few times until you have coordinated it.

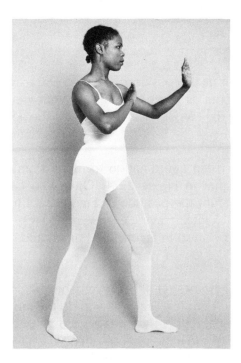

Figure 22.3

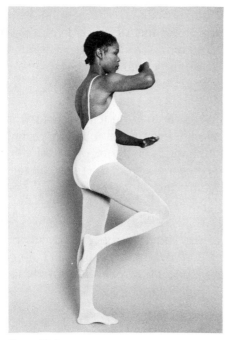

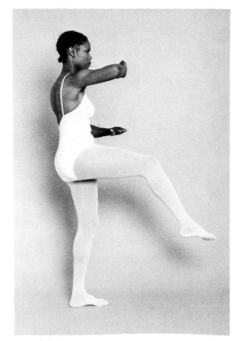

Figure 22.4   *Figure 22.5*

Now, beginning at the position in Figure 22.1 again, move the arms as before, but as you do so transfer your weight to your left foot. Bring your right leg, bent at the knee, to the position shown in Figure 22.4.

Practice arm and leg coordination to move from the position in Figure 22.3 to that in Figure 22.4. Once you can control this, follow through from the position in Figure 22.4 to that in Figure 22.5, with a quick kick. Having executed the kick, sweep your left leg back to the position in Figure 22.3 again and change the arm position.

Once you have mastered the movements beginning with the movement of the right leg, learn how to do the movements beginning with left leg and vary the arms accordingly. Clearly, this is a complex series of movements, but once you have mastered the separate parts, you can put them together and produce movements of great grace and coordination.

The breathing sequence goes like this. Breathe in from the position in Figure 22.3 to the position in Figure 22.4 and explosively push the air for movement from the position in Figure 22.4 to the position in Figure 22.5. Breathe in as you sweep to the position in Figure 22.4 again. Exhale and then continue the cycle.

At first you should do these movements as slowly as possible. This means breathing cycles are slow too, an average performance would be as follows. Positions in Figures 22.3 to 22.4, 3 seconds; positions in Figures 22.4 to 22.5, $\frac{1}{5}$ of a second; positions in Figures 22.5 to 22.3 in 4 seconds; and exhaling as in Figure 22.3, in 5 seconds.

PROTOCOL

Ambrosia: 20 x

Maia: 5 x right leg, 5 x left leg

Ambrosia: 20 x

Protocol Days 5, 6 and 14

Days 23-28

DAY 23: CONSOLIDATION 1

At this stage of the program, improvements in the figure should be well under way. If they are not, you should begin the program again because it means you have not been following it closely enough or working hard enough.

Based on the majority of women who have worked conscientiously, you should be pleased with the results to date. It is now time to consolidate your improvements through a series of protocols in which you think more closely about what you are doing.

PROTOCOL

Read through the theory of stretching again in Day 1. Spend half an hour working on the following, devoting approximately equal time to each.

Persephone (Day 1)

Aphrodite (Day 3)

Venus (Day 5)

Hestia, and massage (Days 6 and 16)

This quiet day should rest your muscles for the hard work tomorrow.

DAY 24: CONSOLIDATION 2

PROTOCOL

Protocol Days 5, 7, 8, and 21

End with massage, Day 6.

DAY 25: CONSOLIDATION 3

After the rigors of yesterday, your tissues need time to recover. Methodically work through Polyxena (Day 12) for 5 minutes, spend five minutes on Phaedra (Day 2), and ten minutes on Hestia massage (Day 16).

DAY 26: CONSOLIDATION 4

Work methodically through the whole protocols of Days 18 and 19.

DAY 27: CONSOLIDATION 5

Today, make a note of the seven exercises you enjoyed most during the program. Put their names and days first described in the following space.

EXERCISE

1.

2.

3.

4.

5.

6.

7.

Now write in one sentence next to each exercise why you liked that exercise. Further, write down against each exercise what it did, and what it does for you in terms of effect on your figure and the pleasure or challenge it gave you. You will be able to answer this easily if you refresh your memory by looking at the photograph. Throughout the program I have urged you to do work in front of a mirror.

These seven exercises can now form the basis of *your* workouts from now on at least twice a week.

DAY 28: CONSOLIDATION 6

Having worked through this program, you may soon never need to work so hard again. You can maintain the gains you have won by using the exercises you chose on Day 27 and by following these four rules.

1. If a part of your figure shows signs of deterioration as the weeks go by, use the book to find a corrective exercise by looking at the contents page and index.
2. Re-read the nutrition advice of the first week from time to time.
3. Check your fat thickness (Appendix 1) every three weeks.
4. Repeat the protocols of Day 21, and good luck.

Appendix 1

YOUR FIGURE, WEIGHT,
AND SKIN FAT THICKNESS

Your skin, far from being a minor component of your total weight, can become one of the major ones if you become overweight because the fat layer beneath the skin can increase in thickness.

On average, a pinch of skin on your body should be about ½ an inch thick. There are slight variations. For instance the pinch on the tummy will be thicker at perfect weight than it is on the forearm. In order to give you an idea of how much excess weight you may be carrying underneath your skin, I have devised the following "pinch" method:

Arm-Chest Measurement

Stretch out your arm with the tape-measure as in Figure A.1. Hold the tape in your outstretched hand as shown in Figure A.2, with the end of the tape at the exact tip of the longest finger and held

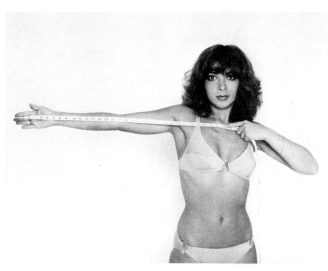

Figure A.1

Figure A.2

Figure A.3

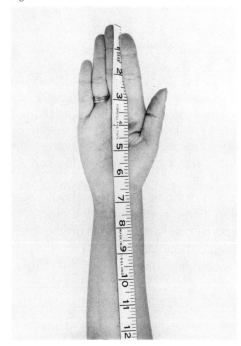

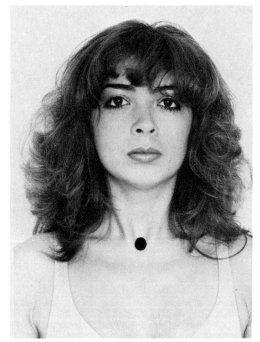

between the first two fingers. Place the tape, stretched taut, at the center of the throat, indicated by the black dot and identified by tensing your neck muscles as shown in Figure A.3. Now read off the arm-chest measurement. In Figure A.1, it is 33 inches. Record your measurement in the following box.

My arm-chest length is_____inches.

My thigh measurement is_____inches.
(5″ from crotch)

My leg pinch is_____inches.

My thigh pinch is_____inches.

My tummy pinch is_____inches.

Total pinch thickness is arm pinch plus tummy pinch plus thigh pinch equals_____inches.

The technique applies mainly and most accurately to women of average physique, that is to say the 5 ft. 6 in., 35 in.−24 in.−36 in. type figure, *but it applies to all body types* more accurately than any other known method.

There are some modifications to be made, however. For taller women, the skin thickness obviously can be a little more. For example, if your arm-chest measurement is 34 in. or more, and especially if you have very large bones, then the fat thickness you can have is about 2 inches all told, without being overweight.

If your total pinch thickness is very near 1½ inches, your weight is about right. If it is only about ¾ inches, you may be getting too thin to have a really healthy figure. For each half inch above 1½ inches, you are overweight.

For example if you have a total pinch thickness of 2 inches, you are ½ inch, so to speak, overweight. If you have 3 inches, you are 1½ inches overweight, and so on.

Look at the American-English chart of ranges. First look at the arm-chest ranges. Find your arm-chest measurement and mark it with a

American–English Chart*

Thigh circum-ference (in.)	ARM–CHEST MEASUREMENT						
	30 in.	31 in.	32 in.	33 in.	34 in.	35 in.	36 in.
16	4½	4½	5	5	5	5	5
18	4½	5	5½	5½	6	6	6
20	5½	6	6	6	6	6½	6½
22	6	6½	6½	6½	7	7	7½
24	6½	7	7	7	7½	8	8

*Increase in weight in pounds for every ½ inch over a total fat skin pinch of 1½ inches.
© Dr. Anthony Harris, 1982.

Metric Chart*

Circumference of thigh (cms)	ARM–CHEST MEASUREMENT						
	76 cm.	79 cm.	82 cm.	84 cm.	87 cm.	89 cm.	92 cm.
41	2.1	2.1	2.2	2.3	2.35	2.4	2.5
46	2.3	2.4	2.5	2.6	2.7	2.75	2.85
51	2.6	2.7	2.8	2.85	2.9	3	3.1
56	2.8	3.0	3.1	3.1	3.2	3.3	3.35
61	3.1	3.3	3.3	3.35	3.4	3.6	3.7

*Increase in weight in kilograms for every centimeter over 4 cm of total fat skin pinch.
© Dr. Anthony Harris, 1983.

check. If your measurement is not exactly shown, pick the nearest. For example if your measurement is 31½ inches, you check 32.

Now look down the thigh circumference column and pick out the nearest value to yours and tick it. Again, if you are exactly between two readings, for example 19, pick the next highest, in this case 20 inches.

Now read down from your arm-chest measurement and across for your thigh (see Figure A.4). Circle the value you find. For example, if your arm-chest measurement is 33 inches and you have a 22 inch thigh, you'll find 6½ pounds given. This means for every ½ inch, fat thickness above 1½ inches, you carry an excess amount of fat of 6½ pounds.

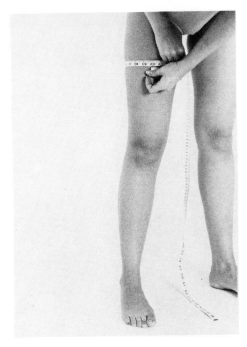

Figure A.4

The charts are very accurate for pinch thickness totals of up to 3 inches. For greater pinch totals, you will *see* from your figure how much it has deteriorated. The charts are for accurate progress monitoring for women who have got out of gross deterioration of body shape.

Appendix 2

SLIMMING DIETS

Having estimated required weight loss, apply these slimming methods as appropriate. The first diet can be used for three or four days, the second diet for a week. In both, variation is the key and you will progress better if you also apply all the principles as established in the first week of the program.

DIET FOR THE OCCASIONAL DAY'S SLIMMING (1100 CALORIES)

This diet is more nutritious than most people's daily fare and gives about 1100 calories a day. The average woman would then have a deficit of at least 1200 calories.

You can use it for up to a week, every other day. Refer to the nutrition section to ensure you apply those principles to the diet.

159

Breakfast (350 calories)

Tea cup measure of cereal (bran, shredded wheat, oats) with ½ cup of milk (should be fresh milk with no more than 2% butterfat to begin. Sweeten with one small banana, orange, slice of melon, or apple. Thin slice of whole wheat toast with marmalade for carbohydrates. Tea or coffee with milk and no sugar can follow.

This breakfast can be varied by varying the fruit and the cereal.

Midmorning Snacks (70 calories)

Tea, or coffee, no sugar, be very sparing with the milk. If hungry, eat an apple, or orange, or banana (small), which each give a maximum of 70 calories.

Lunch (300 calories)

Begin with 4 ounces of plain unsweetened yogurt or melon. For the main course, prepare a boiled egg, or one slice of grilled bacon, or 3 ounces cottage cheese, plus one slice of whole wheat bread. Tea, coffee, or unsweetened vegetable juice can follow.

Late Afternoon Snack

Tea or coffee.

Dinner (350 calories)

Fresh vegetable soup, or melon slice as an appetizer, followed by a main course of an ounce of grilled liver, or one portion of bacon, or a poached or boiled egg, or ounce of grilled steak. Add to this one slice of wholewheat toast with grilled tomato, or green salad (cucumber, lettuce, chopped cabbage, to any amount, with vinegar only). For dessert, one small fruit.

You can use this diet every other day but never more than a week.

SEVEN-DAY SLIMMING DIET

The average person loses up to three pounds of fat in one week on this diet. This diet is balanced in the amounts of fat, protein, and carbohydrates, but even more important it gives high levels of vitamin C and covers the nutrient requirements for minerals and vitamins.

Furthermore, it is a paced diet. For example the amount of fiber is increased as the body gradually accustoms itself to less food, thus alleviating the pangs of hunger.

Each day, you can have only half a pint of milk, and this can be used for cereal, tea, and coffee. You must use 2% butterfat milk. Whenever you feel very hungry and are tempted to break the diet, drink a glass of chilled mixed vegetable juice. Use brand without added salt or sugar. In this diet, you can have a glass of wine where specified.

Having finished the two diets with weight loss of up to seven pounds, revert to your ordinary eating improved by the program nutritional principles of the first week for two weeks, and then if necessary use the diets again as specified.

MONDAY

Breakfast	1 oz. cheese on 1 slice whole wheat bread, 1 grilled tomato Tea or coffee, 2% butterfat milk to taste
Midmorning Snack	Glass of tomato juice, small or large, as desired
Lunch	Main course: 2 oz. grilled steak, 4 oz. boiled carrots, 4 oz. boiled cabbage 1 apple as sweet ½ oz. cheese, 1 soda cracker Tea or coffee, milk to taste
Late Afternoon Snack	1 orange, with tea or coffee
Dinner	Soup: 4 oz. of celery in soup portion. Main course: 2 oz. grilled liver, 2 oz. grilled mushrooms, 4 oz. boiled zucchini 4 oz. melon as sweet Tea or coffee, milk to taste

Last Food of the Day	Tea or coffee, milk to taste

TUESDAY

Breakfast	1 boiled egg, half slice of bread, toasted if desired Tea or coffee
Midmorning Snack	Tea or coffee
Lunch	Glass of grapefruit juice Main course: 3 oz. of steamed haddock, 1 small boiled potato, 4 oz. of peas 1 apple, fresh or stewed, without sugar 1 crisp bread cracker, ½ oz. of cheese Tea or coffee
Late Afternoon Snack	Tea or coffee, 1 water biscuit
Dinner	Avocado pear, 1 tsp. of vinegar and ½ tsp. of olive oil for dressing Main course: 2 oz. of cheese in dish made up of cheese grated over boiled zucchini courgette and mushrooms, 4 oz. zucchini courgette, 2 oz. of mushrooms 1 orange as sweet Tea or coffee
Last Food of the Day	Tea or coffee, 1 water biscuit

WEDNESDAY

Breakfast	1 oz. of grilled bacon, 1 grilled tomato Tea or coffee
Midmorning Snack	Tea or coffee, apple if desired
Lunch	Main course: Cheese salad made of 2 oz. of cheese, 1 oz. of lettuce, 1 medium onion, 1 carrot, half a pepper. Take with 1 slice of whole wheat toast. 4 oz. poached plums, as sweet Tea or coffee
Late Afternoon Snack	Tea or coffee, apple.
Dinner	Soup: Portion of minestrone, made up with any combination of vegetables, excluding potatoes, with ½ oz. of cheese grated on it. (The total weight of vegetables in a portion can go up to 6 oz. and suitable mixtures to make up this amount are cabbage, peppers, carrots, and onions but no pasta)

Main course: Egg and cheese recipe, containing 1 egg, 1 oz. of cheese per portion
1 glass of orange juice as sweet
Tea or coffee

Last Food of the Day Tea or coffee

THURSDAY

Breakfast Boiled egg, half slice of wholewheat bread toasted, ¼ oz. of butter, if required
Tea or coffee

Midmorning Snack Tea or coffee, 1 orange

Lunch 1 cup of bouillon
Main course: 2 oz. of boiled ham, with salad made of 6 oz. of carrots (2 oz.), lettuce (1 oz.), 2 oz. cucumber, 1 oz. onion
1 banana as sweet
Tea or coffee

Late Afternoon Snack Tea or coffee, water biscuit

Dinner This is the half way through the week treat dinner!
4 oz. melon
Main course: 2 oz. of cheese made up of 1 oz. of hard cheese, 1 oz. of soft cheese, to be eaten with green salad (1 oz. of lettuce, 1 medium onion, 1 tomato, 1 green pepper). The treat is in the glass of white or red dry wine.
NO SWEET today, but soda cracker with coffee or tea.

Last Food of the Day Coffee, tea, or cocoa

FRIDAY

Breakfast Now that the calories have been drastically reduced, it is time to expand even more on fiber.
Half a cup of milk, 1 shredded wheat biscuit
Tea or coffee

Midmorning Snack Tea or coffee

Lunch Mixed vegetable juice, made by blending 1 tomato, 1 onion, herbs to taste. Large glasses of this drink can be taken at any time during the diet from

now on when appetite is quickening.
Main course: Egg and cheese sandwich,
made of 1 hard-boiled egg, lettuce leaf,
½ oz. of cheese. Two slices of
wholewheat bread, ¼ oz. of butter.
Tea or coffee—no sweet today

Late Afternoon Snack	Tea or coffee
Dinner	Fresh tomato starter. 1 large tomato, 1 oz. of cheese, radishes, and herbs to taste. Main course: 2 oz. of boiled cod, 4 oz. of steamed spinach 1 orange for sweet Tea or coffee
Last Food of the Day	Tea, coffee, or cocoa

SATURDAY

Breakfast	Juice from 1 orange 2 sardines on 1 slice wholewheat toast (shake off oil on sardines before grilling) Tea or coffee
Midmorning Snack	Tea or coffee, 1 apple
Lunch	Main course: Cheese and wholewheat salad sandwiches made of 2 oz. of cheese, 1 tomato, 3 leaves of lettuce, herbs to taste, 3 slices of wholewheat bread. To be made up as 1½ rounds. Tea or coffee, no sweet
Late Afternoon Snack	1 banana as treat, soda cracker with tea or coffee
Dinner	Treat dinner appetizer: small squares of wholewheat toast (1 slice of bread only) with 1 oz. of toasted cheese, garnish with sprinkled parsley Main course: 1 large potato, with ¼ oz. of butter, 2 oz. of grilled steak, 6 oz. of green salad (2 oz. of lettuce, 1 oz. of cucumber, 1 oz. of green pepper, 2 oz. of celery). Apple as sweet Coffee or tea
Last Food of the Day	Coffee, tea, or cocoa

SUNDAY

Breakfast	4 oz. of yogurt containing sugar 1 orange Tea or coffee

Midmorning Snack	1 crisp bread cracker, tea or coffee
Lunch	Orange juice Main course: per portion, 4 oz. of brown rice, ½ oz. of bacon, 1 tomato, herbs and spices. No sweet today Tea or coffee
Late Afternoon Snack	Tea or coffee
Dinner	End of week special dinner. Main course: 6 oz. of cauliflower, boiled, with herbs and pepper to taste. Grate 2 oz. of cheese over cauliflower, and melt under grill. 4 oz. of beans, boiled, and 1 boiled potato. 4 oz. of fresh fruit salad, made up of 1 oz. each of peaches, apples, oranges and bananas 1 glass red or white dry wine Tea or coffee
Last Food of the Day	Tea, coffee or cocoa

Index